Managing Managed Care

Secrets from a Former Case Manager

Susan Frager

JOHN WILEY & SONS, INC.

New York • Chichester • Weinheim • Brisbane • Singapore • Toronto

Library of Congress Cataloging-in-Publication Data:

Frager, Susan, 1966–
    Managing managed care : secrets from a former case manager / Susan
Frager.
      p.   cm.
    Includes bibliographical references and index.
    ISBN 0-471-35177-6 (pbk. : alk. paper)
    1. Managed mental health care—United States.   2. Psychotherapy—
Practice—United States. I. Title.
    RC465.6.F73   2000
    362.2'0425—dc21   99-37680

To the many people without whom this book would not be a reality, but especially my parents and my husband, for their unflagging emotional and financial support.

To the therapists in the trenches of private practice with whom I am privileged to work every day. Your struggles will remain mine.

To Liz, for giving me the tools (and a few swift kicks when they were most needed) to take those first scary steps out of an abusive environment into a world where dreams do indeed come true.

To Rebekah and Anne, for their friendship, wisdom, and experience.

To my spiritual mentors and healers, Rand Olson, John Reisenleiter, Susan Carol Stone, and Caroline Ziel.

Acknowledgments

"I hate managed care, but it's what enables many of my clients to pay for therapy—I can't resign."

"Just what do they mean by medical necessity anyway?"

"What happens to the personal information on clients that has to be revealed to get authorization?"

"I try never to take managed care clients but it's a competitive advantage to be on the panel. The fees and paperwork are ridiculous, but if I don't stay on the panel, there are enough other therapists out there who will. A low fee is better than none at all."

"Every time I send in one of those reports they lose it. How many times do I have to send one of those things?"

"Their phone systems are a nightmare. I only have 10 minutes between sessions, and it takes 20 just to reach a live voice. They're always putting you on hold and transferring you around."

"It takes 6 months to get paid."

Recognize your thoughts? If so, this book is for you. *Managing Managed Care: Secrets from a Former Case Manager* offers resources and advice for daily practice problems caused by managed care, from the eyes of a former front-line insider. Frustrations and tough choices are certainly endemic to this force which has irrevocably altered the practice landscape, but we do not have to allow ourselves or our clients to be its victims.

The enjoyable part of my job as a case manager at a large managed behavioral health carve-out organization was talking with therapists across the United States. Some were rude, some were angry, but all were competent, hardworking practitioners struggling to survive in a professional world gone mad, just as I was. I learned from my all-too-human reactions to those therapists who were rude and saw first-hand how angry practitioners, right though they undoubtedly are, nevertheless alienate those who might potentially be able to help. These were not fun lessons to learn.

But with the rest, I talked, and listened, and shared, and joked—a lot. Humor is a wonderful antidote to managed care, particularly the obsessive-compulsive need to meet every one of the many financially at-risk contractual promises and QI benchmarks instituted by the powers that be. Most were either next to impossible or else mutually contradictory and just kept getting worse with each new merger.

I began to see that private practitioners of all disciplines need advocates who understand managed care's labyrinthine systems and have the time, patience, and stubbornness to navigate them without giving up. Later, as a practice management consultant to therapists across the country, their struggles with the various managed behavioral care companies, large and small, revealed to me that the similarities across companies were significantly more striking than the differences. Discussions with current and former case managers from various companies, for the purposes of writing *Managing Managed Care*, likewise provided clarity.

It's these case managers to whom I offer my thanks. In addition to case managers, there were also current and former customer service reps, quality improvement, and network department employees, as well as a former member of management, who contributed insights to *Managing Managed Care*. Of this group, I owe the largest debt to Norman Hering, LMFT, the only current or former managed care employee who can be named. His courage in speaking out on the television show *20/20* is an example for us all.

No book of this scope could be written without input from those experts whose names appear repeatedly in various professional publications, and I have many experts in different areas to thank for their time and insights. On the managed care side of things, Erin Somers and Kirk Griffith, PhD, of *Magellan Behavioral Health*, and Jerry Vaccaro, MD, of *PacifiCare Behavioral Health*. Thanks are due, as well, to Margaret O'Kane of NCQA, who understood the need to inform the professional community about NCQA and its standards, the impact of which is only just now beginning to be perceptible in practice life.

Many issues involving managed care now require legal assistance, and there are sympathetic fellow travelers to be found in the legal profession. My sincere thanks to Gayle O'Brien of the New York State Psychological Association, Lee Greenstein, and Joe Sahid, for the time they spent explaining the cases whose implications will affect us all. Then there was Bart Bernstein, a true master of what must surely be considered a fine art among lawyers: the ability to explain legal concepts in a way that therapists can understand and relate to. If we therapists are to continue to do what we do best, then each of us needs a Bart Bernstein to watch our backs.

The voice of the practice community is more than evident in *Managing Managed Care*, and for their time and expertise, I'm grateful to Gordon Herz, PhD, Kathleen Desgranges, LCSW, BCD, and especially to that most prolific of writers and dedicated of activists, Ivan Miller, PhD. Very much in the thick of the issues each month, are John Klein and Candace Glider, editors of *Psychotherapy Finances*, and Gayle Tuttle, of AAMFT's *Practice Strategies*. *Managing Managed Care* would not exist but for their willingness to feature everyday therapists across the country who are creatively engaged in the struggle to keep private practice alive.

My special thanks, as well, to Gayle Zieman, PhD, formerly a managed care executive in his own right and a nationally known consultant to groups taking the plunge and going capitated. Bucking all the trends, Gayle is now back in solo private practice, which to me is a powerful demonstration that no matter how widespread a trend or a fad, some things—like solo practice—are classics that never go out of style. These are lean years, but we'll survive.

There are some truly amazing resources in cyberspace where I've become quite spoiled in terms of getting the news "hot off the presses," as it were, and my favorites are listed as Resources in the Appendix. I'd like to cite Betsy Owens of the NASW e-mail lists, for making my research so much easier, particularly with regard to the "Jane Doe" case. If there was a newsworthy e-mail, chances were good it originated with Betsy. I also owe an immense debt to my cyber-"billing buddies," Linda Walker, Jean Thoensen, Michelle Alswager, and Nancie Cummins, who contributed their comments and opinions for the *"Getting paid: the finances of managed care"* chapter. Linda moderates an extremely supportive and professional forum, a group that made this therapist feel very welcome indeed. Jean, my extra special thanks for your late nights patiently spent hashing over the intricacies and complications of electronic billing, sliding scales, self-pay, "out-of-network" issues, and the setting of fees.

I've saved my most special acknowledgement and heartfelt thanks for everyone at John Wiley & Sons, and most especially for my editor Jennifer Simon, who believed wholeheartedly in the value of what an unknown former managed care employee had to share. Jennifer was there through all the doubts and the growing pains of *Managing Managed Care*, encouraging and yet challenging me to "just write it," but always making sure I remained off the soapbox—not an easy task for a subject like this! Without her patience and guidance, it would truly not have been possible.

A Note about the Use of Terms in Managing Managed Care

It sometimes seems as if no term or concept fully captures the idea one is trying to convey, without either including something that is not appropriate or excluding a group that should be included. With this limitation in mind, I had to make choices regarding the terminology used in *Managing Managed Care*.

The functions of managed behavioral care are currently provided by several distinctly different types of organizations. There are carve-out managed behavioral care organizations, managed care companies, integrated EAP/managed behavioral health firms, HMOs, and Integrated Delivery Systems. The distinctions are certainly critical to a thorough understanding of American healthcare delivery at the dawn of the millennium, but are technical and of little interest to most mental health professionals who are just trying to survive in this brutal age. For the purposes of *Managing Managed Care*, therefore, I chose to use the terms *managed care organization, managed behavioral care organization,* and the related acronyms MCO and MBHO, more or less interchangeably. Where I specifically needed to refer to one type of organization but to exclude the others, I highlighted the distinction at that place in the text.

Pomerantz (1999a) discusses the uncomfortable fact that even the term for this field is in dispute between professionals and managed care. These days word choice can often be a crude but generally reliable indicator of whether or not a speaker or writer is partial to managed care. Professionals, among ourselves, tend to stick to the traditional *mental health, mental health/substance abuse,* or the acronym *MH/SA*. On the managed care side of the fence, the term most often used is *behavioral health*. However, my use of one as opposed to the other should not be interpreted to convey an opinion about managed care. If we are ever to successfully use our knowledge of the current abuses and inefficiencies to transform the current system into a more consumer- and professional-friendly one, then bickering about being "for" or "against" managed care is irrelevant.

Patient versus *client* has recognizable subtleties of nuance and connotation; however, *Managing Managed Care* uses both terms interchangeably to refer to the consumers of our services. I felt it was important to include both terms, if for no other reason than a simple acknowledgement that the readers of *Managing Managed Care* will come from varying backgrounds and disciplines, each of which has its own preference regarding what to call those who benefit from our care.

What do we call ourselves? This was the other major area of terminological decision making I faced in writing *Managing Managed Care*. As a case manager, I had been shaped by my work environment into the regrettable habit of referring to psychotherapists as *"providers."* It's a uniform term managed care has instituted to describe us, and I agree with Shore (1997) that it is degrading. We are highly educated professionals.

Consequently, I've tried wherever possible to avoid use of the term *"provider"* when referring to a mental health practitioner. However, there were times where *"provider"* was the most appropriate word, particularly when referring to managed care practices such as *"provider-profiling,"* concepts such as *"the participating-provider network"* or the managed care company department known as Provider Relations. I used *"provider"* in these instances because it would have created confusion to do otherwise. Names do have power, though, and hopefully we will be able to change these names, as part of the process of transforming the system that created them.

I also made the choice not to refer to practitioners as psychologists, clinical social workers, psychiatrists, marriage and family therapists, or counselors, since these names indicate particular licenses and disciplines. The only way to empower ourselves in the face of managed care is to move beyond professional turf warfare. To achieve this unity, though, I did have to sacrifice a perception of completeness, and thus I want to offer my apologies to any psychiatrist who feels left out by my use of terms such as therapist or psychotherapist. To be exclusive was not my intent; many psychiatrists are legitimate psychotherapists and not merely the drug dispensers that managed care would have them be.

Susan Frager

Contents

1

Life Inside Managed Care

Managed Care 101: Anatomy of a Managed Behavioral Carve-Out Organization

Case Managers

Contrary to common stereotypes, case managers are at least licensed masters' level clinicians, with more than a few doctoral level clinicians doing the same job. Typically, the master's level clinicians have licenses and degrees in psychology, counseling, social work, marriage and family therapy, education, or are licensed/certified psychiatric nurses. Minimum standards of experience are generally 3 to 5 years post-degree (or 1–3 years post-license), with experience in managed care actually much less preferred than experience in direct clinical service.

What Do They Do?   Clinicians work either on an intake line, or with requests for ongoing treatment. Intake-line clinicians work on a *call queue*, the virtual line of phone calls waiting to be answered by "the next available representative." They assess callers for risk, help determine the appropriate level of care, match clients to the appropriate practitioners/services, and authorize the treatment. An integral part of the job of an intake-line clinician is educating callers about how their benefits work. Utilization review case managers work with written data about the client (for example, hospital records or written outpatient treatment reports), and they consult on the phone with clients, therapists, psychiatrists, facilities, family members, and in person with supervisors and psychiatrists about the medical necessity of continuing authorizations for treatment.

Case managers are subdivided into teams based on *account*. Responsibilities on a case management team are typically divided one of three ways:

1. Level of care (i.e., outpatients go to a separate case manager than inpatients).

2. Geography (i.e., all cases in the state of _____).

3. Assigned caseload (i.e., the case manager follows all clients whose last names begin with "A" through "D" regardless of level of care or geography).

This division of responsibilities explains why it's sometimes so hard to find the right case manager.

Very large dedicated teams will often have a further subdivision. For example, there may be several outpatient case managers who are then alphabetically or geographically subdivided. This division of responsibilities explains why it's sometimes so hard to find the right case manager.

Account: Inside managed behavioral care companies, account refers to a contract with an entity to manage the mental health/substance abuse treatment for the "covered lives" of that entity. Accounts can be with employers, unions, city/state governments, Medicaid, or health insurance plans. Also sometimes referred to as a *book of business*.

Dedicated team: Refers to a team that handles only one account.

Case Management Supervisors

As in direct clinical practice, supervisors are available for consultation, help with difficult cases, and advice or decision making in high-risk situations. Supervisors are also in charge of monitoring performance, the team's work-flow issues, internal procedures, and serve on one or more quality improvement committees. They handle complaints from members or practitioners that have not been able to be resolved with the case manager.

When to Use a Clinical Supervisor.   Do not to attempt to bypass the case manager; supervisors will generally not be responsive unless the issue has already been discussed with the case manager and cannot be resolved (Table 1.1). From the supervisor's point of view, this makes sense: If people routinely go directly to supervisors, they will be stuck with all the work. Issues to bring to a supervisor's attention:

- A negative attitude or unprofessional conduct from the case manager.
- Failure of the case manager to return phone calls after a reasonable period of time.

Table 1.1
Fundamentals of Managed Care Relationships

1. The person who answers the phone most likely only has the authority to say "no" to special requests. "Yes" requires someone at a higher level.
2. Arguing with or yelling at someone who does not make the rules and has no power to break them is an exercise in futility.
3. Arguing with or yelling at someone who does not make the rules and has no power to break them is a way to ensure that this person will act as a hindrance rather than a facilitator. Convey understanding of the powerlessness of the individual managed care employee.
4. It is necessary to begin at the lowest level and work upwards; attempts to start at the top will be rebuffed (unless one is a personal friend of the powers that be).
5. Those at the bottom of the managed behavioral care employee hierarchy are continually subjected to complaints about things they are powerless to fix.

- Problems with re-authorization of sessions (i.e., long turnaround time, lost paperwork).
- A request for an exception to administrative policies.

The first three matters can easily be handled with a phone call; get the supervisor's name from the case manager, the operator, or Customer Service. However, a request for an exception to administrative policies must usually be made in writing.

A request for an exception to administrative policies must usually be made in writing.

When making a written request to a case management supervisor, focus on the clinical reasons why the managed care company should grant the request. If it's not a clinical issue, point out the member satisfaction, financial savings, and/or public-relations aspects. Letters that bemoan the tyranny, greed, or unfairness of the managed care company generally don't get the desired response.

Expect the supervisor not to respond personally to a written complaint or request, but to delegate the case manager or even an administrative assistant to respond. They spend much of their time in meetings, so don't be put off by the fact that they are not easily accessible by phone. Leave a voice mail—or put it in writing. However, supervisors generally do respond personally to concerns or complaints regarding case manager conduct.

Do not bother a clinical supervisor about a denial; follow the Appeals process instead (see Chapter 12). Supervisors have no organizational power to overturn a denial, or interfere with a denial process.

Clinical Director

Next up in the clinical department hierarchy is the clinical director, who is responsible for the performance of the case management team with regard to meeting the clinical quality indicators and performance guarantees. Additionally, they monitor the team's adherence to the company "medical necessity" guidelines, and serve as advisors in very high-risk and/or high profile cases. Most companies have several levels of clinical directorships tiered in a hierarchy all the way up to the highest executive levels.

When to Use a Clinical Director. It will rarely happen. If the issue is controversial enough, the case management supervisor will confer with the clinical director or other members of management before making the decision. And, if the issue is considered neither large nor controversial (i.e., a request for a retro-certification), then the supervisor's decision will be accepted as final.

Psychiatrists

Sometimes referred to as *physician advisors* or *psychiatric consultants*, the role of the lower-ranking psychiatrists is to review proposed denials of treatment and in appeals (see Chapter 12). Staff psychiatrists are also expected to conduct internal training on clinical topics, and to serve on quality improvement committees.

When to Use a Psychiatrist. Usually the case managers automatically review certain types of cases, such as inpatients, with the psychiatrist(s). If case managers have questions about other clients for whom review with the psychiatrist is not mandatory, they can consult with the psychiatrist and/or a supervisor. However, nothing can be denied without the review and agreement of a supervising MD or PhD, per the National Committee for Quality Assurance (NCQA) (see Chapter 12). Network therapists are

---

National Committee for Quality Assurance NCQA: Like JCAHO, NCQA is a national not-for-profit organization that issues standards and maintains accreditation programs. NCQA focuses its efforts on the managed care industry (medical as well as mental health) and associated organizations.

free to call the managed care psychiatrist to consult, although in practice it happens rarely. To find the name and extension of the appropriate psychiatrist, ask the case manager or the company operator.

Medical Director

Some companies combine the roles of clinical and medical director, since they are similar in scope, assuring compliance with clinical quality, denials/appeals, and contractual standards. In companies where the clinical and medical director positions are combined, the individual who occupies the position is most often a psychiatrist. A medical director can be over just one team or can be higher up, such as the medical director of all public-sector contracts, or the medical director of the entire company.

Medical directors are in charge of developing "best practices" guidelines, as well as in making revisions to a company's medical necessity criteria (see Chapter 7). They also chair "adverse incident" committees if there is a suicide or some other tragedy, and they have a role on the credentialing committee (see Chapter 3).

When to Use a Medical Director. Medical directors rarely have direct interaction with contracted practitioners, unless there is a suicide or other clinical crisis, or unless a therapist serves on a committee in which there is representation from the contracted network. Interested in participating? Call or write the managed care company's national or local provider relations office. It's not generally an option for a therapist to directly call a medical director to make a request, since they have little to do with the day-to-day authorizations of treatment or other administrative issues.

Interested in participating? Call or write the managed care company's national or local provider relations office.

Customer Service Representative

Sometimes these individuals or departments are variously known as Member Services, Patient Care Coordinators, Care Coordinators, or Intake Service Representatives. They are always available on call queues and typically are the first "live voice" reached through the menu of options. Customer Service representatives have a wide variety of functions, and their purpose is often to get as many calls as possible handled without necessitating transfer to other departments or individuals. Don't underestimate the utility of the customer service reps, even though they are not clinicians.

Don't underestimate the utility of the customer service reps, even though they are not clinicians.

Getting to the Right Place.   Like case managers, member service personnel are generally divided into teams based on account. How can one be sure of reaching the right team? Call the number on the client's benefit card. Most mistakes happen when clients say, *"I have Managed Care Company Y,"* and the therapist, office staff, or billing service uses the number they have on file. Although eventually callers will be routed to the correct team, it's much quicker—and eases the frustration factor—to call the dedicated number for the client's employer or health plan. If you get transferred, be sure to ask for the correct number to dial the next time.

The Importance of Using the Right Account Team: Accounts have different benefit limits, copayments, precertification requirements, deductibles, and so on. Talking to the wrong team is a setup for being given the wrong information which creates a mess later.

When in doubt about who to contact regarding a particular matter, customer service is always a good place to start.

When to Use Customer Service.   When in doubt about who to contact regarding a particular matter, customer service is always a good place to start. Some reasons to call a customer service representative include:

- Eligibility and benefits verifications (see Chapter 13).
- Benefit information (copayments, deductibles, annual limits, etc).
- Certification questions (end-date extensions, certification/authorization numbers, confirming what was certified).
- Changing CPT codes, start/end dates, frequency, or other features of certifications. (At some companies, any changes to certification might require case manager permission.)
- Registering or precertifying treatment. (At some companies, clients may be required to precertify with an intake clinician.)
- Verification that outpatient treatment reports were received.
- To obtain names of participating professionals/facilities.
- To verify the network status of a particular clinician/facility.
- Claims questions.
- To make a complaint. Customer service will generally take the information and route it to the appropriate employee for follow up.

Not sure whether what you need is handled by case management or customer service? When in doubt, start with customer service since they are more immediately accessible by phone.

Customer Service Supervisor

The supervisor(s) in charge of the customer service representatives are responsible for monitoring the call volume, making sure that the staffing is adequate to meet the demands and that relevant telephone-service benchmarks are met. Customer service supervisors also monitor the phone conversations, reviewing tapes or listening "live" to make sure that the employees are meeting the needs of the callers and handling the interactions in a professional manner. They serve as important sources of information if a customer service representative does not know the answer to a particular question. Sometimes, customer service supervisors are also responsible for the initial handling of complaints received by members and/or practitioners.

When to Use a Customer Service Supervisor. Complaints about behavior, negative attitude, or mistakes made by a customer service representative should be directed to the supervisor. For every interaction with any kind of managed care employee, it's vital to record the name of the employee, the date, and the nature of the conversation in the client's chart. This information will be needed in the event that a supervisor needs to be contacted, if the employee has made a mistake that results in a denied claim or some other problem.

Claims Department

The main responsibility of the claims department is to process claims (technical term: *adjudicate*). Like case managers and customer service representatives, claims processors are also most often subdivided into teams based on benefit plan or employer, with the goal being to achieve greater familiarity with a smaller number of benefit plans, thus improving accuracy in claims payment.

Where Do I Call to Get Claims Problems Fixed? Follow the telephone prompts. Depending on how the managed care company has arranged itself organizationally, the option "if you have a question about claims" will either lead to customer service or to claims.

It's vital to record the name of the employee, the date, and the nature of the conversation in the client's chart. This information will be needed in the event that a supervisor needs to be contacted, if the employee has made a mistake that results in a denied claim or some other problem.

Don't They Pay Claims?   The large national managed behavioral care carve-out companies, with covered lives in the millions, do pay claims, but the smaller, regional managed care companies, group practices, and/or integrated delivery systems that have capitated contracts and some managed care functions may actually not pay claims themselves. When the claims are not paid in-house, network professionals usually are unaware of the fact. They are still instructed to submit their claims to such organizations, just as they would to the larger companies. What then happens is that the claims are re-priced (the full fee is adjusted to the contracted rate) and sent on to the insurance company for payment. When this is the arrangement, there is no need for a full-fledged claims department, and callers inquiring about claims may be referred to the claims payor.

Network/Provider Relations

Provider Relations or Provider Services is a department made up of individuals on a call queue who answer questions about fees, contracts, joining/resigning the network, (re)credentialing, and making requested changes, such as a change of address, to a therapist's record or file.

Network Development and/or Network Management, usually under the same organizational umbrella, is distinct in function. They handle (re)credentialing, primary source verification, specialty credentialing, recruitment, following up on complaints that have to do with network

Table 1.2
Using Provider Relations

- Call them to get instructions regarding changing an address, phone number, tax ID, etc. (Note: The request to change information usually has to be received in writing.)
- For answers to questions about contract terms.
- To verify the current contracted fees for the various CPT codes/procedures.
- To manage referral volume (i.e., requesting a period of inactivity, how to receive more referrals).
- Questions about joining or resigning from the network.
- Question or confusion about network status.
- Questions about credentialing or recredentialing packets.
- When licenses and malpractice insurance are renewed, send copies ASAP to Provider Relations—call to get the address.
- If the contract is for a group practice, questions about adding or deleting additional practitioners to/from the contract.

members' conduct, and (in conjunction with the Quality Improvement Department) site visits and provider-profiling.

Using Provider Relations/Network. Provider Services is an important resource; most of the large managed behavioral care companies have specific toll-free numbers for professionals to call; some companies divide the United States into regions and have regional Provider Relations centers. It's a good idea to keep note of the correct number(s), although most of the phone systems are set up such that dialing a number listed on a client's card will usually have a Provider Relations phone menu option (Table 1.2).

Quality Improvement (QI) or Quality Assurance (QA)

Quality departments have two main functions:

1. Monitoring/ensuring the company's compliance with contractual performance guarantees.
2. Monitoring/ensuring the company's compliance with the standards of NCQA and other accrediting organizations such as JCAHO and URAC.

Large, influential benefits purchasers have always been able to customize their managed behavioral health plans in order to improve quality. Before NCQA became involved in the attempt to regulate and standardize managed behavioral health, companies such as IBM and Digital Equipment were working side-by-side with the large integrated EAP/managed behavioral health firms to design customized packages (Astrachan et al., 1995; Oss & Clary, 1998). Several of these packages' features were later integrated into NCQA's standards for all managed behavioral health-care. The states picked up the idea when they turned to managed care for Medicaid behavioral health. Iowa, Michigan, Massachusetts, and Colorado, for instance, now specify contractual performance guarantees for the managed care companies that handle their Medicaid behavioral health business (*Managed Behavioral Health News*, 1998b). Performance guarantees are routinely offered as sales tactics, as one way for purchasers to differentiate among the large carve-out behavioral health managed care companies who are offering more or less the same price.

A *performance guarantee* highlights a specific quality or service indicator and contractually guarantees, through financial incentives, a certain

A performance guarantee highlights a specific quality or service indicator and contractually guarantees, through financial incentives, a certain level of performance.

level of performance. Performance guarantees are handled either by means of withholds or rebates. In the first case, the purchaser retains a predetermined amount of money and does not pay the managed care company until the target guarantee is demonstrated. In the rebate method, the managed care company owes the predetermined sum of money back to the customer if the target is not met (Bengen-Seltzer, 1998; *Managed Behavioral Health News*, 1998b). Performance guarantees occur in all aspects of the operation of managed care companies. Each of the measures listed in Table 1.3 is known as a *quality indicator*.

The Regulatory, "Report-Card" Approach to Quality.   NCQA's standards govern most aspects of life inside managed care. Like JCAHO, NCQA's surveyors go on-site to measure how the organization performs on each of its standards, using interviews with staff and various types of documentation as source material. The surveyors are concerned with measuring the company's internal performance on the standards, and if compliance is deemed sufficient, the company receives accreditation. NCQA also uses a tool called HEDIS® (Health Plan Employer Data and Information Set), which profiles companies on a carefully selected set of medical and behavioral health clinical, service, satisfaction, and utilization indicators. HEDIS can be considered NCQA's version of performance guarantees; there is typically a fair degree of overlap between common contractual performance guarantees and HEDIS indicators, which are also the basis for the "report cards" published in the attempt to help consumers choose between various HMOs.

HEDIS can be considered NCQA's version of performance guarantees; there is typically a fair degree of overlap between common contractual performance guarantees and HEDIS indicators.

Performance Measures for Managed Behavioral Healthcare Programs (PERMS), are published by the managed behavioral care trade group, American Managed Behavioral Healthcare Association (AMBHA). PERMS, like HEDIS, is a set of specific measures on which companies are rated, and its indicators are also similar to contractual performance guarantees, because it is developed by representatives of the same companies who sign the performance guarantees. PERMS, unlike HEDIS, is strictly concerned with behavioral health.

There's no shortage of other behavioral health plan performance measures. JCAHO has its own set of indicators, called ORYX. The government bureaus, SAMHSA and the Agency for Healthcare Policy and Research, use their own measures as well. There are other smaller foundations and consulting firms that use their own standards and tools to measure and compare health plan performance.

Table 1.3
Sample Common Performance Guarantees*

Service Indicators:

- Telephone Service: Callers to the member line will reach a live voice in at least 25 seconds 98% of the time. There will be a less than 3% overall abandonment rate.
- Claims Processing Time: Clean claims will be paid in 30 days or less 95% of the time.
- OTR Turnaround Time: Ninety-nine percent of outpatient treatment reports will be reviewed within 9 working days of receipt.
- Member Satisfaction: The rate of member complaints will not be more than 6% of the total member population. Ninety-five percent of member/patient complaints will be responded to within 2 working days, and 100% of complaints within 4 working days.

Network Indicators:

- Accessibility: Routine clients will have an initial appointment within 6 calendar days 95% of the time, and within 8 calendar days 100% of the time.
- Adequacy: No more than 5% of all claims paid on an in-network benefit basis will be paid to a professional with an ad-hoc or temporary network status.

  Ninety-five percent of members calling for referral are given the names of at least 3 in-network therapists within 20 miles.
- Specialties: In areas of at least 500,000 total population, there will be at least 3 network professionals with specialized credentials and/or specialty training in each of the following areas: children/adolescents, marriage/family therapy, eating disorders, substance abuse, neuropsychology, and geriatrics.
- Cultural Competency: In urban areas of greater than 1 million total population, there will be at least 2 network professionals of the gender, ethnic/racial/cultural background of the client's choice 85% of the time.

Clinical Indicators:

- Substance Abuse: Ninety-five percent of clients diagnosed with either a primary or secondary substance abuse disorder or who are dual diagnosis, will be referred to applicable 12-step self-help groups as part of their treatment plan. Ninety percent of clients receiving treatment for substance abuse issues for at least 6 months will exhibit a 2-day-per-month reduction in absenteeism at work.
- Major Depression: At least 90% of clients with a primary or secondary diagnosis of moderate or severe major depression will receive psychiatric evaluation for medication.
- Utilization: Inpatient re-admission rate will be less than 2% after 120 days, and less than 5% after 365 days.
- Sixty-five percent of clients referred to EAP will resolve problems in EAP without necessitating referral to outpatient psychotherapy using managed mental health benefits.
- Continuity and Coordination of Care: Ninety-six percent of all clients discharged from inpatient or partial hospitalization programs will have initial outpatient follow-up appointments within 5 working days of discharge.
- There will be consultation with primary care physician in at least 90% of cases.

*Target percentage measurements used in the sample indicators are to be regarded as examples only. The target levels of performance in actual contracts is proprietary information.

Quality improvement works with information-systems staff to config-
ure the managed care company's computer system so that the statistics
necessary for measuring the quality indicators will be captured. Reports are run on a regular basis for interpretation by members of the QI
department, who work with other staff as needed, usually in the form of
committees, to improve performance and prepare for accreditation au-
dits/site visits. QI also has a hand in developing outcomes measurement
instruments, "best practices" and medical necessity guidelines, updating
treatment report forms, and various documentation standards. QI's
major interface with the Network Department concerns the speed and
accuracy of the credentialing process, newsletters and other communications to the entire network, and refining *provider-profiling* measurement
procedures (see Chapter 3).

Using QI—and Its Usefulness.   Network practitioners do not have direct
interaction with members of the QI department, but their work becomes
part of the data collection. There would be no reason for a therapist to
contact a QI staff member, and QI does not directly contact members of
the network. If there is a need to inform one particular therapist about a
specific issue, a case manager is usually directed to make the contact.

*Whether
performance
guarantees,
accreditation, and
report-card
methods actually
ensure quality,
and are worth the
sums currently
spent, is an open
question.*

Whether performance guarantees, accreditation, and report-card methods
actually ensure quality, and are worth the sums currently spent, is an open
question. Often millions are spent to achieve accreditation (Mihalik,
1998). One independent auditor of managed care plans, has concluded
from his audits that 45 to 50 cents out of every premium dollar goes to the
administration and profit of the managed care company (Wrich, 1998).
The Hay Group (1998) demonstrated that the value of behavioral health
benefits fell 54 percent over a 10-year period, although employer spending
to purchase benefits remained about the same. Although it is clear that
this is money that could be paying for treatment, purchasers of benefits
expect documentation of quality; reform proposals will be faced with the
challenge of identifying clinically effective, cost-effective, and less bureaucratic methods of quality measurement.

Appeals

When treatment is denied, clients and their therapists have the right to
appeal the decision (see Chapter 12), and the Appeals Department is responsible for the efficient handling of appeals.

Account Management and Sales

Sales or marketing staff respond to requests for proposals (typically referred to as RFPs) from employers, health plans/insurers, state and city governments, and so on—anyone who is offering a benefit package that will include mental health/substance abuse. They identify what the customer needs in a behavioral health benefit package and negotiate a deal. This is the process by which the structure of the mental health/substance abuse benefits, the price, specific contractual performance guarantees, limits, and what is and isn't covered is determined.

Carve-out refers to the widespread practice of separating the behavioral health benefit plan from the medical benefits, and administering each plan independently. *Carve-in* behavioral health benefits are administered as part of the medical plan. The decision to carve out or carve in is entirely up to the purchaser of the benefits. It is not decided by managed care companies. The system of carve-ins and carve-outs has resulted in a frustrating and time-consuming process of having to untangle who does what among the various contracted and subcontracted corporate entities—each time there is a new client wishing to use insurance to pay for therapy.

After signing the contract, the managed care company assigns one or more *account managers* or *account liaisons*. Their job is to ensure that whatever is promised is delivered, and to this end they work closely with higher level clinical operations and quality improvement staff to monitor services and make improvements.

Navigating the Managed Care Company Phone System

Using the operator, unfortunately, isn't necessarily faster than selecting the most plausible-sounding phone menu option. There are rarely more than two or three operators on duty at any one time, and they're always busy, so be prepared to sit through as many as 50 rings.

Sometimes there is an option that allows the caller to connect to a particular individual by entering the name on the keypad until the system recognizes the name of the employee. It's a waste of time searching for an extension number through an automated employee name directory.

What if you spell the name wrong? What if that employee has left the company? And if the system merely routes the phone call instead of giving out the extension number, it's the same dilemma next time a call needs to be made.

A few companies' phone systems send calls to a group voice mail or receptionist after waiting a certain length of time:

> You've reached the customer service division for ChoiceBank, at UltraCare Behavioral Health. Call volume is higher than expected today. Please leave a message after the beep with your name and number, and someone will return your call as soon as possible.

Calling back repeatedly until someone takes the call generally works.

They do this because *abandonment rate* (the percentage of people hanging up while on hold) is a commonly-used performance guarantee (see Table 1.3). Don't leave a message; if they're too busy to answer the phone, then they're going to be too busy, at least for the foreseeable future, to call back. One of the facts of life on a call queue is that there's never any end to the calls. Calling back repeatedly until someone takes the call generally works. Or, find an operator. I've generally found that if I modulate my tone such that my frustration is combined with a friendly *"please help me, I'm overwhelmed,"* attitude, operators are very willing to keep me on the line while they page someone to pick up the phone.

Are there times to call when it is easier to get through? Call volume is always unpredictable. Instead, bad times to call are when there are likely to be fewer employees answering the phones. Times to avoid: the first hours after opening on Monday mornings, the one or two hours just prior to closing on Friday afternoons, the lunch hour, and the entire day after a major holiday or 3-day weekend.

After Normal Business Hours

Managed care companies do have clinicians available 24 hours per day, seven days per week. Some companies may have a few after-hours customer service reps available as well. Psychiatrists rotate on-call duties in case there is an after-hours denial. That is the extent of the staff on duty at night, on weekends, and on holidays, and consequently, they are limited in the types of calls they can handle. After-hours coverage is for two purposes only: (1) clinical crisis and (2) emergency precertification/ referral. Obvious, but I've taken calls from people angry about denied claims at midnight, on the Fourth of July, and on Thanksgiving Day. Use the following list as a guideline:

What can be handled after-hours?

- Clinical emergencies (suicidal callers, etc.).
- Hospital admissions.
- Request for critical incident stress debriefing (CISD).
- Referral requests for EAP or outpatient therapy.
- Initiating an expedited appeal (see Chapter 12, Denials and Appeals).

Wait till the next business day for:

- Checking on denied claims.
- Checking on receipt/status of outpatient treatment report.
- To extend an authorization end date or "good-through" date.
- To request a back-certification.
- Benefits verification/eligibility check.
- Detailed questions about benefits (i.e., does the plan cover EMDR?).
- To review with a case manager for continuing authorization (any level of care).
- To check on network status/ask questions about participating-provider contracts.
- To register a complaint.
- To request the name of one specific employee in any department who can fix your problem or answer your question.

After-hours clinicians may not even be in the same state as the service center that handles the daytime calls; phones can be forwarded anywhere. With smaller managed care companies, it can be even more confusing because the after-hours function might be subcontracted out. Some integrated delivery systems and capitated group practices have a hospital-based telephone triage unit. After hours, there's no way to know where the phone is ringing on the other end.

Why can't they answer benefit/eligibility questions after hours? It depends on how the managed care company has arranged its after-hours operations. Subcontracted companies aren't always given access to the benefit and eligibility information system. And there may be too many different benefit plans to ensure accuracy of answers to benefits questions. As an

After hours, there's no way to know where the phone is ringing on the other end.

Calling the appropriate team during the daytime maximizes the likelihood of receiving correct benefit/eligibility information.

after-hours crisis clinician, my team was responsible for over 800 EAP and/or managed care accounts. Calling the appropriate team during the daytime maximizes the likelihood of receiving correct benefit/ eligibility information.

Interacting Positively with the Phone-Queue Employee

Understanding the employee's situation can be empowering for therapists who feel completely powerless when having to work with managed care. This includes provider relations and customer service; it doesn't refer only to clinicians. Managed care companies are noisy, frenetic environments. The managed care employee might not be consciously aware of the multiple demands on the physiology of his or her attention, but it does require sustained effort to focus concentration on the caller. Calls of a similar nature tend to blur after a while; from the employee's perspective, it's natural to feel like a broken record and forget that the caller currently on the line hasn't heard you say the same thing again and again.

Managed care companies often place a great deal of money at-risk for meeting their telephone-service performance guarantees (see Table 1.3). As call volume increases, jeopardizing performance levels, so does the stress of the employees taking the calls. There may be other expectations of management that increase employee stress. One clinician interviewed, who had worked in three different positions at two major companies, indicated that there was a certain number of calls per day that intake clinicians were required to handle. Management would post updated statistics each hour, and employees' job performance was measured by how close they came to the benchmark number of calls. "I felt it was counterproductive insisting on a certain number of calls, because that meant the calls were too quick and there was no time to follow up [*to make sure everything was done right the first time*]. This would increase problems and increase calls [*in the long run*]."

Be clear about the information that must be obtained prior to hanging up. Having an agenda for the call enables one to take control of the conversation.

Have an agenda. Be clear about the information that must be obtained prior to hanging up. It may actually help to have a checklist in writing, particularly when verifying benefits. Having an agenda for the call enables one to take control of the conversation. Getting flustered or angry doesn't help and allows the managed care employee to continue with his or her abruptness, impatience, and so forth. Take responsibility for getting your needs met (doesn't this sound like something we often say to our clients?).

How Does the Employee's Stress Typically Show Itself to Callers?

- Abruptness.
- Rapid talking.
- Uses technical insurance jargon; difficulty explaining in everyday words for caller to understand.
- Uses prewritten scripts.
- Talks louder than normal (the same phenomenon seen when trying to make the deaf or those who speak a foreign language understand).
- Impatience with questions or caller's difficulty understanding.
- Frequently interrupts the caller.
- Doesn't solicit questions or verbal clarification from the caller.
- Appears to be in a hurry to get off the phone.
- Does not ask if there is anything else they can do for the caller at the end of the conversation.

Build documentation time into the call. The live voice on the other end of the line is required to document everything, no matter how trivial. Sometimes, if computer systems are old and/or if there is a merger underway, the employee may be required to document the same information in several places in the system, or using more than one computer platform. But sometimes supervisors who perform silent telephone audits score down if they can hear the employee typing during the call. Employees may instead be expected to make notes, and then enter the information into the system when not on a call, increasing the risk that documentation of the calls, promised changes to certifications, and/or new authorizations can lag behind or be forgotten altogether. The old cliché, *"if it isn't documented, it didn't happen,"* is the number one rule for working with managed care, and sometimes it's also *"If it isn't documented CORRECTLY, it didn't happen."*

Help yourself and the managed care employee at the same time. Say clearly into the phone, if you don't hear the employee typing, *"I can take as much time as you need to enter my request into the system."* Or even, *"I'd like to request that you enter a note into the system while we're still on the*

Say clearly into the phone, if you don't hear the employee typing, "I can take as much time as you need to enter my request into the system."

phone together. It's not that I don't trust you, I just want to make sure that [the claims get paid, the client's authorization gets entered into the computer, etc.]." Managed care employees not only understand this, they're grateful for it. If the supervisor is auditing, it gets them off the hook. It can help break the barriers and create a brief feeling of rapport. Depending on how they are treated, powerless employees at the bottom of the managed care hierarchy can be either facilitators or hindrances.

If the employee says the computers are down, call back. Yes, it's a hassle. But it's worse if the employee forgets to enter the information into the system when the computers come back online and claims get denied as a result.

It's an unwritten rule of managed care: supervisors know that things slip through the cracks, and the "proof" of originally having called is to be able to furnish a name and a date.

Get the employee's first and last name. Ask him or her how to spell it. If the employee responds by saying, "We're not allowed to or we don't give out our last names," don't be upset or flustered. Simply apologize and ask for the first initial of their last name. Most employees will give it; they know and understand why this question is being asked. It's an unwritten rule of managed care: supervisors know that things slip through the cracks, and the "proof" of originally having called is to be able to furnish a name and a date.

Extensions aren't generally considered necessary for purposes of "proof." An extension number is for the purpose of dialing that specific employee directly at a later time. Employees on an automated call distribution system are considered to be interchangeable. It sounds demeaning, but think about it from the perspective of a competent team member. If he or she gave out a personal extension upon request, he or she would get a lot of direct calls, because therapists would want to avoid less competent peers, and the workload would eventually become unfairly distributed. In addition to skewing the workload, taking calls directly from the outside rather than from the phone queue is a no-no for call queue employees: rightly or wrongly, supervisors may assume that these are personal calls.

Asking for an extension is a good habit to develop.

But since it's not always possible to tell whether a particular employee works on a phone queue, asking for an extension is a good habit to develop. When asked for an extension, sometimes a call queue employee will give out the extension number of the call queue itself. The call queue extension is good information, because it's a time-saver. One of the first options on most automated voice menu systems is usually: "If you know your party's extension, dial that extension now." Dialing the call queue extension number circumvents having to listen to the rest of the menu.

Some employees will refuse to give an extension or say that they don't have one. This may not be true, but don't antagonize a managed care employee over this issue.

Voice Mail Etiquette

Automated call distribution systems eliminate the need to leave voice mail, which is found primarily when working with utilization-review case managers.

Andrew Reviewer is listening to his 40 voice mails shortly after his arrival at work at GenRUs Behavioral Health on a Monday morning:

1. October 14, 3:45 PM. <beep> "Hi, this is Connie Cook, and I'm calling about my son James. He's 14 and failing all his subjects. I talked to you last year requesting testing, and nothing was done, and this year James absolutely must be tested. . . . Please help, I don't know who else to call, and his therapist says she won't do the testing unless you approve it. We've scheduled the testing for Tuesday, so I need to hear from you on Monday at the latest. Please call me back at (555) 111-2234. Oh, my husband's social security number is 321-12-1234 and he works for Precision Engineering."

2. October 14, 4:01 PM. <beep> <deep sigh> "You never answer your phone. It's impossible to get to talk to one of you guys. This is Dr. Porter from Richmond, Virginia. You have my treatment plan and I need to know whether Daisy Doe is certified so I can continue seeing her. My number is (666) 987-0123."

3. October 14, 4:16 PM. <beep> "Hi Andrew, I'm calling about my client Liz Tyler, social security number 123-45-6789, and my name is Dr. Jonathan Livingston in Hartford. Anyway, the authorization ran out last week and I'll send you one of those reports, but in the meantime could you just give me one session so I'll get paid for seeing her tomorrow? Liz is still depressed, still taking Prozac, and we're exploring why she has trouble being assertive with men. Please help me out, ok? I promise, it will never happen again. My number is (999) 567-8901. If you can't approve it, please page me at (999) 567-8911 and we can review it over the phone. Thanks!"

Each of these voice mails is ineffective in some way. As a direct result, Andrew will be unable to fulfill the callers' requests, leading to further frustration on their part. Here's why:

1. Connie Cook is setting herself up, because her expectation that Andrew will approve testing might not be realistic (see Chapter 11).

Also, she left the message late on a Friday afternoon, for Andrew to be getting it first thing Monday morning, and she's telling him he needs to call her back that day. That might just not be possible—and then what does Mrs. Cook do? Cancel the testing? Or go ahead with it, and challenge any claims denial, saying she called ahead of time?

2. Dr. Porter starts off by complaining. Not a great way to build an effective collegial relationship. But more importantly, what's Daisy Doe's insurance ID number and who is the employer/what is the health plan? How is Andrew supposed to know where to look for her certification? What will most likely happen is that Andrew will forward the message to an assistant, who will have to call Dr. Porter back to get Daisy's insurance information, frustrating him further by managed care's "incompetence."

3. Dr. Livingston gives Andrew a way to find his client's record in the computer, and he's friendly, but is setting himself up for a denied session. He's hedging with having to complete a treatment report, hoping that Andrew will: (1) be able to call him back in time; (2) be able to connect with him; and (3) be willing to review over the phone. Giving a pager number is a good idea, but it doesn't guarantee that a busy case manager and a busy therapist will connect. Furthermore, Dr. Livingston has left clinical information for Andrew on the voice mail. It implies that Andrew should just "be a good guy" and use that information to justify authorizing the session. At some companies, that might not be a problem, but at others, case managers are very clearly expected to refuse—or even ignore—all such requests. Andrew might just forward the voice mail to an assistant requesting that Dr. Livingston be contacted and told to fill out a treatment report, because if he agrees to Dr. Livingston's request "just this once," where's the incentive for the doctor not to do it again?

Use the 10 rules of voice mail etiquette in Table 1.4 as a survival guide. Following them will allow for a better experience; it's a win-win situation for both the therapist and the case manager—and, ultimately, the patient.

Paging Etiquette

Case managers like to keep it fairly quiet that they can be paged. If misused, it can be a hindrance rather than a help to getting things done. A

Table 1.4
10 Rules of Voice Mail Etiquette

1. Always leave the client's full name and the insured's social security number or case/authorization number (*leaving the client's social security number, if the client is not the insured, is useless*).

2. Always leave a complete phone number—including area code—where you can be reached for return calls. The line should be answered by voice mail or an answering service if you are not available.

3. Always identify the name of the insured's employer or benefit plan.

4. Always state clearly and precisely what you need the case manager to do.

5. Don't leave clinical information unless you have prior permission or unless the outgoing message says that it's OK to do so and that the voice mail is confidential in nature. Even if the voice mail says it's OK to leave clinical information, voice mail is not necessarily considered an acceptable substitute for a written outpatient treatment report or live telephone review.

6. Give the case manager several good times to reach you over the next two business days.

7. Speak slowly and clearly, spelling your last name and/or the client's if appropriate. Repeat the phone number.

8. Don't expect that the case manager will be able to adhere to a tight time frame. If you need something immediately, page the case manager or make your request of another live voice who can either help you himself or herself or will alert the case manager.

9. Don't leave a voice mail for a clinician about a denied claim or other nonclinical issue that is more easily dealt with by a live voice in the Customer Service Department.

10. Don't yell at the person from whom you're requesting help!

colleague of mine was once paged no less than 5 times in a single hour by the mother of the client he was reviewing for residential treatment.

Having said that, there are times when it is necessary to page a case manager. To page, find an operator, and request to be put on hold while the case manager is paged. The operator generally will check back in a few minutes if the case manager doesn't immediately respond; simply ask the operator to keep trying. Company operators are very useful individuals. Because of the nature of their jobs, they get to know the names of virtually every employee. If the case manager cannot be found, request to speak to another case manager, or a supervisor.

To page, find an operator, and request to be put on hold while the case manager is paged.

Interacting with All Managed Care Employees

Some tips for day-to-day situations:

- *Don't personalize the impersonal.* When talking to an employee, reserve the pronoun *you* to mean only the employee. When referring to the managed care company in general, rather than the employee

When talking to an employee, reserve the pronoun you to mean only the employee.

COMMON ABUSES OF THE PAGING SYSTEM

Want to stay out of the case manager's bad graces? Don't do any of the following:

- Page the case manager for a telephone review of outpatient treatment because you don't have time (or don't want) to do a written treatment plan. *(As the saying goes, failure to plan on your part does not constitute an emergency on my part.)*
- Page the case manager for a new client who needs precertification ASAP. Use the intake line, it's actually just as fast.
- Page the case manager about a nonclinical matter (claims, end date extensions, retro-certification, etc.). Use customer service. Or, if directed by customer service to the case manager, leave a voice mail.
- An outpatient client who needs to go to the hospital. Use the Intake line; they might be able to authorize it. The Intake clinician will direct callers to the case manager if his or her approval is needed.

APPROPRIATE USES OF THE PAGING SYSTEM

- You have a pre-arranged telephone appointment with the case manager but the line is busy.
- To do a review of a client who is inpatient and needs to stay inpatient, or has need of some other procedure on an emergency basis.
- To obtain precertification for follow-up care for a client who is being discharged from the hospital.
- You have left several voice mails without a return call.

in particular, use the company's name, or say *the company*. Using *you* when referring to the company as a whole implies that the individual speaks for, agrees with, and has personally implemented, each and every abusive or bureaucratic policy and practice. Not only is this false, it's interpersonally alienating.

- *Don't complain about fees or other managed care policies the employee is powerless to fix.* Don't make comments, joke, or complain about policies, paperwork, or low fees, unless (1) there is a relationship developed with the managed care employee; and (2) the employee indicates being OK with complaints (usually signaled by the employee making comments, jokes, or complaints). Managed care employees who are psychologically invested in the system will feel threatened and react negatively to comments about these topics—even comments which were intended as humorous, or as just plain statements of the truth.

- *Make a clear, specific request.* What do you need from the employee? Don't make them work hard just to clarify their role in your request. If it's not clear what the request is, then you may be venting.

- *Keep the focus on the client's treatment plan and needs.* Fairly self-evident, but not always as easy as it sounds. Managed care is frustrating.

2

Getting on
Participating-Provider Panels

A few years back, if a therapist wanted to be on managed care networks, all she or he had to do was call. An application would be sent, which the therapist could take an unlimited amount of time to complete. This is no longer true. Managed care companies are now more choosy about who they let in largely because of two global trends: Managed care steadily increased its market penetration to where it is a rare client who has insurance that is not "managed" in some form or other. Second, the behavioral health professional population has also drastically increased (see Chapter 14).

Closing the Panels

Maintaining a network is a significant operating expense. There are the costs of (re)credentialing, primary source verifications, staff, mailings, trainings, and so on. The managed care companies, however, consider that the actual dollar cost of maintaining one network professional is proprietary information and unanimously refused requests for estimates when contacted.

Maintaining the smallest number of professionals possible on a network is in the best economic interests of the managed care company.

Network development people have been known to say that one of the reasons for closing the panels is that *"our providers get angry if we open it up to too many people. If we do that, they won't get enough referrals."* Possibly, but if the wishes of contracted therapists dictated managed care company policy, there wouldn't be so many complaints about low fees. Ultimately, the major reason for closing the panels is that maintaining the smallest number of professionals possible on a network is in the best economic interests of the managed care company. Concentrating the referrals to as small a number as possible improves a managed care company's ability to measure outcomes, to conduct *provider-profiling* analyses (see Chapter 3), and increases the economic dependency of the network professionals on the managed care company.

The Formula for a "Full" Network

The most widely-used internal measure is that for all but the most rural locations, patients should have to drive no longer than 20 minutes or no further than 25 miles to access outpatient treatment. But what does this say about what's reasonable to expect from a carve-out managed behavioral health plan in terms of a minimal degree of choice? "Reasonable," unfortunately, has not been defined in terms of hard numbers by the industry, nor by the NCQA.

NCQA does not set minimum standards for network density or degree of choice (1998, 2000). Managed care companies are allowed to set their own internal standards for the number and density of professionals on their network, and are not required to reveal the nature of these standards to their members. Managed care companies are allowed to specify which professional disciplines and license types they will and won't accept into their networks. Nor is there a standard requiring managed care companies to give the consumer a minimum number of choices among professionals on the network. Nor is there a specific standard defining the maximum driving distance or time the consumer must spend to reach the nearest network practitioner; this is left to the determination of the managed care organization.

Even though the managed care companies consider their exact network density formulas to be proprietary information, it is possible to make some estimates. Mills (1997) reports an academic study on the oversupply of behavioral health professionals. This study indicated that about 70 professionals per 100,000 members of the general population would be a balanced proportion (see Chapter 14). Or, per 1,000 "covered lives," this would be 0.7 (i.e., 1) practitioner.

Predictable Patterns of Network Development

In general, managed behavioral care companies will staff their networks such that, if available in the area, there will be at least one male and one female practitioner from each of the three most common disciplines (psychiatry, psychology, and clinical social work), within a 25 to 30 mile radius. In more populated areas, companies will add professionals to make sure that specialties such as child/adolescent, substance abuse, marital/family, and so on are represented. Wherever possible, companies then try to diversify their networks further to include professionals in different neighborhoods, those with more specific clinical specialties, and those with varying linguistic, ethnic/cultural, and racial backgrounds.

Kirk Griffith, senior vice president of Clinical Network Management, Magellan Behavioral Health, shared his observations on network development: "There is a market-driven conflict and tension with regard to appropriate numbers of providers. Some employers believe more is better, and so push for large networks. But there's the cost issue, and also a challenge with regard to managing care and identifying outcomes."

Managed care companies will offer purchasers the chance to make their own choices regarding the types of professionals they will accept as "in-network."

Contract-specific requirements often influence the choice of who will be allowed to participate on the network. Managed care companies will offer purchasers the chance to make their own choices regarding the types of professionals they will accept as "in-network." This is how professionals may end up as "participating" for some accounts, but as "out of network" for others. Although it's not as common as it used to be for masters' level clinicians to be excluded, the occasional benefit plan will specify "*Ph.D.'s only.*" And there are still many that will not accept LPCs or licensed marriage and family therapists.

Caveat: NCQA.   There is one feature of network selection that actually is covered by NCQA standards. If the covered population has special needs or demographics, the NCQA requires that the MBHO choose professionals for the network that match the needs/demographics of the population being served (NCQA, 2000, QI4.1). For example, a Medicare HMO should make sure that there are adequate numbers of professionals with geriatric specialties. However, the cultural competence clause seems to be fairly vague and may be difficult to prove for accounts with diverse membership.

Should Managed Care Be Allowed to Control Access to Qualified Practitioners?

Some states have passed laws mandating insurance carriers and managed care companies to accept any professional who wishes to join the panel, is willing to accept the discounted fees and other policies, and who has the published minimum credentials. Hence the name of these laws, "any willing provider."

"Any willing provider" laws aren't, economically, to the advantage of the managed care companies. To continue to meet the standards they have set for themselves through the NCQA, "any willing provider" laws force companies to spend an unknown amount of money in (re)credentialing (see Chapter 3). Companies also lose money in claims payments, if they are no longer able to deny or reduce payment because of a professional's out-of-network status. Not surprisingly, the managed care companies' trade association, the American Managed Behavioral Healthcare Association (AMBHA), released a position paper in 1997 arguing against "any willing provider" laws using the familiar rhetoric of ensuring positive quality and outcomes while controlling costs.

"Wannabes"

If managed care lobbies succeed in blocking "any willing provider" legislation from being enacted, or if the companies are able to get around loopholes in laws already in force, what about the rights of the individual psychotherapist to practice his or her profession? Therapists who meet the credentialing standards, and who are willing to accept the fees and policies of the managed care companies, are essentially being told *"we think you're superfluous in your area."* High and low alike on the inside blame practitioner oversupply, and point the finger at the graduate schools.

Casting blame about the oversupply of behavioral health practitioners, the policies of universities, or the greed of managed care companies doesn't solve the problem, which is clearly one of unequal power. From a strictly legal standpoint, it is an anti-trust violation for therapists to attempt to collectively bargain with, or boycott, the managed care companies for better conditions. However, the largest managed care companies control a sizable portion of the market. Not being on a participating-provider panel means that a therapist is significantly less able to compete for the population of clients who wish to use their insurance benefits. It has yet to be determined legally if the managed care companies are actually interfering with the free market for their "covered lives" in terms of practitioner choice. Watch for new developments over the next several years, as more self-employed healthcare professionals, spearheaded by physicians, indicate a desire to affiliate with unions, as new legislation is enacted at the state level, and as anti-trust lawsuits begin to be heard in the courts.

Therapists who meet the credentialing standards, and who are willing to accept the fees and policies of the managed care companies, are essentially being told "we think you're superfluous in your area."

Not being on a participating-provider panel means that a therapist is significantly less able to compete for the population of clients who wish to use their insurance benefits.

Questions to Consider before Investing the Time and Energy Needed to Break into a Closed Network

When companies say their network is closed, they mean that the internal formula specifying an acceptable number of professionals per discipline per number of "covered lives" in the area has been met, and that they would prefer not to take on the extra expense of another network participant. Therapists who wish to join a closed panel must convince the network department that their addition will be cost-effective and enhance the overall quality and variety of the network. Is the effort worth it? Consider:

Therapists who wish to join a closed panel must convince the network department that their addition will be cost-effective and enhance the overall quality and variety of the network.

1. What is the saturation of potential clients with insurance plans managed by this company in this area?
2. What kind of clients typically have this insurance plan?
3. How many clients have chosen to go elsewhere in the last 12 months because I was not on this particular insurance/managed care panel?
4. Does this insurance plan have out-of-network reimbursement?
5. If the insurance plan does have out-of-network benefits, do I have to precertify? Submit treatment reports?
6. What does the company pay in-network clinicians? How much of a reduction is it from my full fee?
7. Assuming I choose not to join, does my practice offer enough other incentives to persuade clients to use their out-of-network benefits or pay out-of-pocket (better confidentiality, lack of paperwork, no need to precertify, highly regarded in community, clinical specialty, more convenient because of location, wait times, etc.)?
8. Consider your specialties, training, experience, community reputation, languages, ethnic/cultural background, and client population. Is at least one of these unique enough in your community to make you seem a "must-have" to the managed care company?
9. How does the company treat its network members? Are the company employees accessible by phone? What are the paperwork requirements? Do they pay claims quickly? Talk to colleagues on the network.
10. Is being on this panel so important that I am willing to invest the time and energy into attempts to join the network that might not be

successful for 12 to 18 months? Energy and time to engage in marketing a practice are both finite resources. It's best to allocate them where they will do the most good.

The answers to questions 1 and 2 can be obtained through companies that specialize in this kind of profiling (see Appendix). These statistics are expensive, but they may be useful tools. Consider splitting the expense with colleagues. Sometimes provider relations representatives can give out facts and figures on how many "covered lives" the company has in a particular city or state, but many companies consider it proprietary data.

If the Answer to Question 10 Was Yes . . .

Don't give up. Sooner or later it will happen. Eventually, if for no other reason than attrition, there are openings on managed care panels. Managed care companies lower the fees, people get tired of the paperwork, therapists resign, retire, change careers, move out of the area, and so on. Companies also are always bidding on new business, and "we have a special network, tailored to your needs" is a common sales tactic. New business in an area generally creates at least a few openings on the participating-provider network.

Send an updated resume/vita with letter of interest every 6 to 9 months. It's like applying for a job at a company you'd really like to work for. Just as human resources departments keep resumes on file, so do network development departments. They purge their files every so often, which is why persistence is important. Keeping the company updated signals eagerness to work with them, and also ensures that the information on file remains current. Some companies who receive interest letters with a vita enter the clinician's name into their database as being interested in joining the network; this is one way to get on the company's mailing list.

Keeping the company updated signals eagerness to work with them, and also ensures that the information on file remains current.

Try to get the name of a specific person. If this isn't possible, send the materials anyway, addressed to "Manager, Network Development." Do not let the *"our panel is closed"* answer act as a deterrent to sending a vita and interest letter. If you don't let the company know about yourself and your practice, how will they know of your interest and existence when an opening comes up? Call to follow up 2 to 3 weeks after sending the resume/vita and letter of interest. If you were able to get a specific name, ask to speak to this person. Treat this person according to the fundamentals of managed care relationships mentioned in Chapter 1.

Do not let the "our panel is closed" answer act as a deterrent to sending a vita and interest letter.

The Letter of Interest

Start by expressing interest in participating on their network. Briefly demonstrate your knowledge of them, then go on to show why they need you and what you can do for them. Keep it to one page. The letter should spotlight those parts of your practice most likely to appeal to managed care companies. The goal is to have the network development manager say to him- or herself: "We really need this practice/therapist on our panel!"

The goal is to have the network development manager say to him- or herself: "We really need this practice/ therapist on our panel!"

Elements of Practices That Appeal to Managed Care:

- Location (near large concentrations of "covered lives").
- Easy access for clients who must use public transportation.
- Office(s) that are fully accessible to disabled clients.
- Evening and weekend appointment hours.
- Multidisciplinary/easy access to clinicians of other disciplines.
- Formalized agreements with network professionals of other disciplines for referral purposes (*let the company know that the psychiatrist's office schedules your clients ASAP*).
- Twenty-four hour access (*specify: pager, answering service, etc.*).
- Able to return phone calls within an hour or two.
- Able to schedule new clients immediately (same or next day).
- Specialty areas that are in short supply.
- Offer therapy groups on a regular basis.
- Ability to conduct therapy in a foreign language or sign language.
- Therapists from varying ethnic/cultural backgrounds.
- Computer information systems for tracking patients, outcomes, billing/scheduling, and so on.
- Integration/cooperative and close working relationships with medical professionals.
- For practitioners specializing in children/adolescents, cooperative and close working relationships with the school system.
- Willingness/ability to perform outcome measures and other quality assurance tasks.
- Hospital privileges (*even "allied professional" or "visiting" privileges are useful, because they demonstrate a willingness to treat clients on an interdisciplinary basis, and assure continuity of care regardless of the client's treatment setting*).

Not all of these elements are necessarily the province of the large group practices. No practice is going to have every single element or be all things to all people.

Don't be afraid to be creative. Network development departments receive hundreds of these letters each week. Find a way to make it stand out—or it will get tossed onto a pile with the others (see Table 2.1). The idea is to make a creative and attractive professional presentation that sets you apart from the rest.

As with a resume or vita, make sure the interest letter is free of typographical and grammatical errors and is printed on quality paper, preferably a letterhead.

Get feedback. After writing the letter, put it aside for a day or two. Then try to reread it from the perspective of a busy network development employee who receives hundreds of these in a week. What stands out? Get someone else to read the letter. Ask them what catches their eye. After reading the letter, does the practice seem like a must-have, or is it only "ho, hum"? If you know anyone who works for a managed care company, regardless of their position, ask them for their opinion. This letter is the first and only impression that the managed care company

Table 2.1
Creative Ideas for a Managed Care Interest Letter

Include a folder with:

- Articles you've written.
- Handouts on clinical specialty topics.
- Brochures.
- Flyers for current therapy groups.
- A copy of your practice newsletter.
- A map to the office.
- A photograph of yourself (or group photograph, if a group practice).

People with more high-tech skills might consider:

- A video introduction to the practice and/or walkthrough of the office.
- Sending the information on computer disks.
- E-mailing the interest letter with the resume/vita as a file attachment (since no one currently sends interest letters via e-mail, it's a way to attract attention).
- Including the information in the style of an Internet Web page, and sending it on a disk.

has of you and your practice, so make it as positive and professional as possible.

Ad Hoc Status: The "Back Door" to the Network

An ad hoc (or temporary provider status) means that for one particular client, a nonparticipating therapist is treated as a member of the network and will be paid at in-network rates, but his or her name hasn't been permanently added to the panel.

An ad hoc (or temporary provider status) means that for one particular client, a nonparticipating therapist is treated as a member of the network and will be paid at in-network rates, but his or her name hasn't been permanently added to the panel. The ad-hoc practice is expensive for a managed care company. It requires more of a case manager's time. It also requires the involvement of network, who must check the requested therapist's credentials, negotiate a rate, add the name to the participating-provider and claims databases, and process a temporary contract. In the competition for business, furthermore, some managed care companies have signed financially at-risk "network adequacy" performance guarantees (see Table 1.3). Then there's the extra money spent paying claims at in-network rates.

A Touchy Subject for Case Managers

Although the case manager typically is the recipient of these requests to add therapists to the network due to a "special situation or circumstance," he or she has no power to grant them. Every case manager interviewed from a Big Five company indicated that either a supervisor or provider relations/network needed to approve ad hoc requests. When, as is often the case, the request is denied, the case manager is then usually the bearer of bad news. Former case manager Norman Hering said, "I hated having to tell someone that their request was denied . . . I had no control over things, and people would give me a hard time."

Today, an ad-hoc request is likely to be approved only given one or more of the following circumstances:

Characteristics of the Client

1. The client is a VIP and specifically requests the out-of-network therapist.
2. The client makes enough noise that the managed care company decides not to risk complaints/the client complains to his or her HR department, union leadership, or benefit administrator, who intervenes.

3. The client's employer switched managed care plans during the course of the client's treatment. The new managed care company *should* ad hoc on the basis of continuity of care, at least for the duration of the current episode of treatment.

Deficits in the "Participating-Provider" Network

4. There is no network therapist within the specified driving distance of where the client lives. (Some companies are even stricter—if the client lives in a remote area but works in an adequately staffed one, they will argue that the client must see a panel member near the work location in order to receive in-network benefits.)

5. The out-of-network therapist is of a gender, ethnic, or racial background not represented in the network within 20 to 30 miles, or speaks a language spoken by no other network participants within 20 to 30 miles.

6. All in-network therapists of a needed specialty are 30+ miles away from the out-of-network therapist.

Characteristics of the Client and Deficits in the Network

7. The available network professionals can't be used due to dual roles and/or conflicts of interest (the network therapist and the client are neighbors, belong to the same church, the network therapist is the parent of the client's child's best friend, the network therapist is treating the patient's ex, etc).

Proceed with caution and diplomacy. Using the ad hoc to gain entry to a closed panel can be very effective, if the temporary network status is granted. However, the tendency is to expect clients to take responsibility for obtaining the therapist's ad hoc network status, and earlier literature on managed care (Browning & Browning, 1996) even made this recommendation. Nothing could be more wrong, from a strategic point of view as well as from an ethical one.

Browning and Browning's (1996) thinking is that a client requesting the ad hoc has more of a chance of getting it to go through than the out-of-network therapist. The client has the ability to complain to his or her boss, human resources department, union leadership, or insurance plan administrator. This is all true. Managed care companies, no matter how powerful they seem, are accountable to their customers. The client, through his or her employer, union, or insurance plan, is a customer. The therapist, regardless of network status, is not.

Managed care companies, no matter how powerful they seem, are accountable to their customers. The client, through his or her employer, union, or insurance plan, is a customer. The therapist, regardless of network status, is not.

Vincent Vango, employed in the art department of a large ad agency, wanted to see Erica Adler, PhD, who was not part of GenRUs Behavioral Health's panel in New York City, where in her block alone there were about 20 names on the network. She was starting to lose business as a result. Dr. Adler had been recommended to Vincent Vango as a specialist for bipolar disorder. However, when Vincent called to precertify, the GBH employee gave him the names of 5 other psychologists in the same two-block area who had listed the same specialty.

Vincent called Dr. Adler back, reluctantly concluding he needed to see one of the network psychologists. Dr. Adler, annoyed at losing yet another prospective patient to managed care and convinced that she would be a better choice for Vincent than any of her colleagues, explained to Vincent that his illness was serious, and that GBH should be responsible for offering him the best possible care. She suggested he schedule an appointment, then call to request that she be added to the network.

Vincent did as Dr. Adler suggested. The case manager warned him that his request had little chance of success, and in the end the request was denied. By then, Vincent had started treatment with Dr. Adler, and did not want to switch therapists.

Dr. Adler, attempting to empower Vincent, then suggested he complain to human resources about GBH's lack of respect for his situation. Afraid now that he was accumulating a large bill, Vincent kept on fighting, which caused his symptoms of irritability, anger, grandiosity, and sense of entitlement to worsen.

Ethically, is this justifiable? It's not as if Vincent had been seeing Dr. Adler for years. He is a new client and could just as easily have chosen a psychologist from the list. One could even argue the possibility that Dr. Adler engaged in an act of malpractice by implying that none of her colleagues were appropriate to treat Vincent; she manipulated him into seeking treatment that would not be benefit-covered without a fight, when he clearly wanted his insurance to pay. That fight, and the worry over the bill, was contributing to the worsening of his presenting symptoms. There is absolutely no guarantee, even with all Vincent's efforts, of a favorable final outcome. All the managed care company has to do is say that there are enough panel therapists, and give him the choice between changing to a network member or using his out-of-network benefits, assuming his plan has them.

Ethically, Dr. Adler would have been on safer ground if she had simply explained to Vincent the advantages in working with her (i.e., greater confidentiality), leaving Vincent to make the final decision about whom to see and whether to fight with the managed care company over adding her.

Keep the boundaries clear. If the client wants to undertake the work needed to pursue an ad hoc, make sure the treatment record clearly shows that the client is calling and/or writing letters because he or she wants to. Clients do use the argument that requesting an addition to the network causes stress and a worsening of the original problem(s), so ensure the case notes reflect that the client—not the therapist—is the originator of the stress.

Case managers are often instructed to use their clinical skills to ferret out who is really behind an ad hoc request. Let's say Vincent continued to make a lot of noise. It's very likely the case manager's supervisor would suggest a call to Dr. Adler to determine why she is clinically the best choice for Vincent. After all, temporary providerships must be justified. But what is Dr. Adler going to be able to say, other than that they have already begun treatment? This isn't a very persuasive argument, since Vincent knew Dr. Adler was not a network participant when they began. Nor is Dr. Adler going to get anywhere by denigrating her network colleagues' skills.

Negative comments to a case manager about professional colleagues never create a favorable impression, and aren't effective. If therapists are suspected of unethically using clients for their own ends, the company will feel perfectly justified in refusing the ad hoc request.

What should a therapist say if the request to be added truly was the client's idea and the managed care company calls, inquiring? Take the stance that you are flattered that the client thinks so highly of you, you certainly are well-qualified to treat this client, and you would appreciate the professional opportunity to be able to work with this managed care company. Also, convey a clinical understanding that the client may be operating from an oppositional or entitlement perspective that is potentially more reflective of his or her Axis I or II issues than anything to do with the nature of your practice or your skills as a therapist.

Ethical and Effective Ways to Request
Temporary In-Network Status

Make sure there is justification for the request, using the circumstances listed earlier as guidelines. First, have the client request a complete list of the network practitioners in the area to determine whether there are

Clients do use the argument that requesting an addition to the network causes stress and a worsening of the original problem(s), so ensure the case notes reflect that the client— not the therapist— is the originator of the stress.

What should a therapist say if the request to be added truly was the client's idea and the managed care company calls, inquiring?

Complete lists are hard to get; however, clients who utter the magic words "I'm thinking about requesting that Dr. Out-of-Network be added for my case" generally will provoke a managed care employee into sending the entire list.

The client should be prepared for the possibility that the ad hoc request may be denied and alternative payment arrangements will need to be made.

inadequacies in the network. Complete lists are hard to get; however, clients who utter the magic words "I'm thinking about requesting that Dr. Out-of-Network be added for my case" generally will provoke a managed care employee into sending the entire list. The company will use the complete list, including the names of therapists that would otherwise never be given out for the purpose of referrals, to prove that their network is adequate. Also, find out if the client's benefit plan has out-of-network benefits. Discuss the pros and cons with the client of forging ahead with a temporary providership request.

Starting therapy before the ad hoc is approved is very tricky. The client should be prepared for the possibility that the ad hoc request may be denied and alternative payment arrangements will need to be made. Dr. Adler's unethical behavior certainly extended to conveying the expectation that the ad hoc would be granted if Vincent just fought hard enough. The "they'll give it to you if you just make enough noise" philosophy may require louder and more persistent complaining than many clients may be willing to undertake. However, is it ethical or appropriate to make the client wait two or three weeks to begin therapy while the issue is being decided? A case manager and/or supervisor can give a no answer the day of the request or the next day, but if the client decides to appeal, this process could take several weeks.

Whatever is decided, make sure the client understands the circumstances and the risks. As a method of both self-protection and informed consent, consider outlining all the options in a letter to the client. Have the client sign the letter and keep a copy in the chart.

Taking the Next Step

Once a temporary in-network status is granted, it's not likely to be made permanent unless the ad hoc was granted due to deficits in the network. Political ad hocs do go through and the out-of-network therapist may even greatly impress the case manager, but this doesn't change the fact that adding a therapist is an expense the managed care company isn't willing to undertake. But, there's never any harm in asking!

When talking to the case manager and/or the provider relations employee who processes the ad hoc, politely express thanks on behalf of the client and your interest in being a permanent part of the network. Do this verbally at the beginning of the client's treatment. Then, as the client is getting ready to be discharged, write this in a letter to the

Provider Relations Department. Make sure that treatment reports and other documentation are up to standard, and always return phone calls promptly. The same factors that cause in-network clinicians to be highly rated as "managed care friendly" are even more crucial for professionals wishing to join the network on a permanent basis.

Frequent Fliers

Multiple ad hocs usually signal to a managed care company that they should add that particular professional to the network. It's usually cheaper to offer a participating-provider contract than to repeatedly go through the bureaucracy and expense of completing an ad hoc. However, joining the network may not be the best course of action. If there truly is no one else in the area, therapists have the power to obtain better reimbursement rates (see Chapter 14).

Completing the Application

> Dina Troy, LCSW, receives a participating-provider application from UltraCare Behavioral Health. On it is a large red sticker saying, "Application must be returned within 30 days from date of receipt or it will be presumed that provider is not interested in joining the network at this time. To start the application process over after 30 days, contact Provider Relations at (800) 888-8888."

These warnings are a result of today's crowded panels. Typically, managed care companies don't go to the trouble and expense of sending out applications unless:

1. There are openings in the therapist's geographic area.
2. The company has a closed network, but has prescreened the therapist (via the interest letter or prescreening application), and is in need of that therapist's specialties or demographics.

Those "return-in-30-days-or-else" warnings serve as a kind of disclaimer to therapists, and should be interpreted literally. In other words, the companies are saying, *"You're being graciously invited to join our otherwise closed network—respond today!"* From a recruitment standpoint, tight turnaround times for applications mean that the Network Development Department can retain a degree of control over the influx into the network.

Those "return-in-30-days-or-else" warnings serve as a kind of disclaimer to therapists, and should be interpreted literally.

Dot All the Is and Cross All the Ts

Don't leave anything blank. It may sound obvious to Dina Troy, LCSW, that she doesn't have hospital privileges, not being an MD, but it's not so obvious to the credentialer who processes her application. Many hospitals have Allied Health Professional privileges that can be granted to non-MDs. These applications are written to be as generic as possible across all disciplines and the entire United States. So, it would be advisable for Dina to write "none" or "N/A" in that space. Trivial? Undoubtedly. But the person or team who processes applications doesn't have time to contact applicants about each and every unclear or blank answer. Call provider relations with any questions about applications, no matter how trivial they might seem.

The person or team who processes applications doesn't have time to contact applicants about each and every unclear or blank answer.

Specialties on a Managed Care Network Application

No issue is more anxiety producing to therapists when applying for managed behavioral healthcare or EAP panels. This huge corporate entity has an impact on the financial success of a practice. No wonder therapists tend to approach the specialty portion of the application as if it were a *make-you-or-break-you* encounter!

Our concerns generally sound like this:

- If I call myself a specialist, then I'll get boxed in. I won't be able to enjoy the variety of clients that keeps my practice fun.
- I specialize in PTSD, but how do I prove that to the managed care company? How do they define specialist?
- I've done a lot of work in substance abuse, but I don't have a substance abuse credential. Do I list myself as a specialist if I don't have the credential? It's not fair to have to pay money to have an extra credential in order to be considered a specialist.
- How many is too many specialties? If I put too many, they'll think I'm Jack of all trades, and master of none. Yet if I don't put enough, they'll see me as not qualified.
- All these specialties are clinically related to each other; why do they have Phobias listed separately from Anxiety?

Nonclinical, network management professionals are generally baffled as to why therapists routinely treat the specialty portion of the application as if it were a trick question. Network management departments think of *specialty credentialing* as a way to profile the network professionals, making it easier for case management, intake, and customer service to match a client with a therapist who is likely to be effective with that client. It is considered a quality improvement function, in fact. Another use for specialty credentialing is to determine how many, and what kind, of professionals the managed care company still needs to recruit to their network for a given geographical area.

However, there are no guidelines at this time that uniformly define what credentials or experience are necessary in order to be considered a specialist in a given area. NCQA (1998, 2000) Credentialing and Recredentialing Standards do not address the issue. Thus, each managed behavioral care company is currently free to define specialties as they see fit. Making it even more confusing are the numerous mergers and acquisitions, which can result in each geographical region, account, or corporate division having its own standards defining what constitutes a "specialty" in a given clinical area.

Each managed behavioral care company is currently free to define specialties as they see fit.

Sometimes the applications include the definition of specialist used by that particular company. For example, "Applicant must have 2,000 hours of documentable training and clinical experience in order to be considered a specialist." Wherever the company has defined what they mean by specialist, adhere to that definition. The problem is that few of us after any number of years of practice have our training and experience broken down into numbers of hours.

Sometimes there is guidance from applicable state law(s). For example, certain states have regulated specialties such as marital/family therapy and substance abuse. Therapists who live in states where a particular specialty is regulated should only call themselves specialists if they possess the applicable state credential or license.

National professional associations sometimes offer credentials that can be helpful in defining specialties. For example, it is generally accepted that someone who meets the American Association of Marriage and Family Therapy (AAMFT) standards for a clinical member can claim the marital/family specialty, even if that therapist's state has no marriage and family therapist license. But what about more specific specialties, such as depression, or treatment of individuals with dissociative disorders? The large national professional organizations don't generally offer such specific credentials.

Specific Practice Area Credentials

There are many smaller clinical societies, offering credentials for narrower fields of practice, such as a specific disorder, or certification in a particular technique or theoretical approach. But it's far from a popular idea; credentials cost money to obtain and maintain. With managed care having spent the last several years cutting reimbursement rates, it's adding insult to injury in the eyes of the therapist community to even imply that these credentials are needed—or will someday be needed—to claim a particular practice specialty.

Professional credentials and associations are an accepted way of informing the public that, unlike Lucy in the *Peanuts* cartoon, a particular therapist didn't just hang up his or her shingle and begin dispensing advice. Furthermore, professional associations generally mandate adherence to a code of conduct, provide continuing education opportunities, and advocate for their members on relevant issues.

The Common Consensus Approach

Answer questions about specialties according to what therapists in your particular clinical and geographical areas would say is a specialist.

If there are no guidelines from the managed care company, the state, or a professional association, pretend a trusted colleague in the community is making a referral to you. What would he or she tell this client about your specialties? That's all this really is. You are telling the managed care company what you do best, so they can pass this information on to the client. The difference is in the area of trust. Consider actually asking one or two such colleagues for their feedback. Ultimately, the best advice is to answer questions about specialties according to what most reasonable, experienced therapists in your particular clinical and geographical areas would say is a specialist.

The Right Number of Specialties to Claim

Be careful not to list more than two or three specialty areas on an applications.

Each managed care company is different in the nature of its application, policies, and procedures. But be careful not to list more than two or three specialty areas on an application, because the people processing applications may be instructed not to look past the second or third one listed (*Psychotherapy Finances*, 1998).

All too often, the list of specialties will look something like this:

Please check the following which you consider to be your specialty areas:

____ Children	____ Brief therapy
____ Adolescents	____ Psychoanalysis
____ HIV/AIDS	____ Suicidal clients
____ Addictions	____ Relationship difficulties
____ Geriatrics	____ Veterans' issues
____ Autism/pervasive developmental disorder	____ Anxiety
	____ Psychopharmacology
____ Divorce	____ Chronic physical illness
____ Depression	____ Psychological testing
____ Obsessive-compulsive disorder	____ Schizophrenia
	____ Cognitive-behavioral therapy
____ Personality disorder	
____ Ethnic minorities	

Just ask a clinician what's wrong with this list, and you'd get an earful. It mixes diagnoses, client populations, and treatment modalities. Some diagnostic categories are quite specific (Autism, HIV/AIDS), and others are hopelessly general (Personality Disorder—as if all people with a diagnosis on Axis II were the same!). Client populations can be misleading in their generality as well (do all children and ethnic minorities have the same issues?). Plus, how does one choose between a treatment modality such as cognitive-behavioral therapy and a diagnostic category for which it is usually effective (such as depression)? Managed care companies who send out applications such these really should have one of their in-house clinicians act as an advisor.

It's tempting, but don't correct the list. Just pick the two or three most relevant areas, keeping these strategies in mind:

- *Avoid choosing overlapping diagnostic categories.* The advice to limit the number of specialties selected means that therapists should choose carefully, making each specialty count. To choose both Anxiety and Obsessive-Compulsive Disorder (OCD), for example, wastes a choice because OCD is an anxiety disorder. In the case of more than one choice being given for a diagnostic category, select the broadest option. Referring clinicians will know that a specialty in anxiety means a specialty—or at least proficiency—in OCD.
- *Take care with categories that are too broad.* Addictions, for example. How many substance abuse specialists treat gambling or sexual addictions? Sometimes eating disorders are treated according to an addiction model, but they certainly aren't the same as either substance abuse or gambling. Therapists whose specialties are best represented by a much broader choice on an application's checklist should consider writing the more specific specialty in the margin. For instance, a therapist completing the sample application would check "addictions" but then clarify "substance abuse only." The same applies to large groups of client populations.
- *Avoid the obvious tricks: Modalities not approved of by managed care.* Why are they asking about psychoanalysis? This is a managed care application. Well, some companies have been known to do this kind of thing as a way to determine whether therapists really are "managed care friendly."
- *Avoid the obvious tricks II: Specialties usually not covered by managed care plans.* Relationship difficulties? It may be a specialty area, but it's a waste to mark it on an application, since managed care will never cover V-Codes for the various relationship problems. In these days of crowded panels, choosing a specialty like this will detract from the perception of need for that applicant on the managed care company's network.

3

Credentialing and Network Management

Carla Rogers, EdD, received an application from UCBH, which she completed and returned. The application had included a contract, so Carla assumed she was now in-network. Three weeks later, she began seeing a UCBH client, Bobbi Bentley. However, Bobbi's claims were paid as out-of-network. When Carla called, she was told it was because her credentialing was not complete. Provider Relations confirmed receiving Carla's application and explained she would know she was active when she received a welcome packet. When Carla asked how long that would be, she was dismayed to hear the answer, "3 or 4 months."

After the Application Is Submitted: The Credentialing Process

What could possibly take so long? Once an application to join the managed care company's network has been submitted, it goes to the Network Department for *credentialing*, the process of checking the applicant's degree, licensure, work experience, specialty training/certifications, privileges, malpractice coverage, and so on, to assure that everything meets the standards of the managed care company.

As performed today, credentialing is a laborious, time-intensive, and expensive process. Zieman (1998) estimates the cost of credentialing a single clinician as being in excess of $200. NCQA (2000, CR 3) specifies that the following information, at a minimum, be primary source verified:

1. License for independent practice at the highest licensure level available in the state.

Credentialing is the process of checking the applicant's degree, licensure, work experience, specialty training/ certifications, privileges, malpractice coverage, and so on.

2. Valid degree; the educational or professional program must have been accredited at the time of graduation.
3. History of malpractice claims/lawsuits or lack thereof.

These items are also subject to primary source verification, if they apply to the practitioner:

4. Active DEA license and prescription privileges are current and unsanctioned.
5. Board certification.

Primary source verification is the process of verifying credentialing information directly with the university, state licensing board, malpractice insurance carrier, or other entity that issues credentials.

The primary source verification, the process of verifying credentialing information directly with the university, state licensing board, malpractice insurance carrier, or other entity that issues credentials, is what takes so much time. It's usually 3 to 6 months from the time an application is submitted until the time the therapist becomes active as a participating-provider. There are also other required credential checks that managed care companies must make on each professional applicant (NCQA, 2000, CR 5). The relevant state licensure board or the National Practitioner Data Bank must be checked for any record of complaints or other disciplinary action. The malpractice insurer must furnish a complete claims history, if applicable. Additionally, plans must verify if there has been any history of sanction or questionable conduct.

Attestations

These are a series of yes/no questions, usually found right before the signature page of the application. Signature indicates that the information is complete and correct to the best of the applicant's knowledge. Attestations are required by NCQA (2000, CR 4) in these areas:

1. "History of loss of license and felony convictions."
2. "History of loss or limitation of privileges or disciplinary activity."
3. The applicant is not currently using illicit drugs.
4. "The reasons for any inability to perform the essential functions of the position, with or without accommodation."
5. Malpractice insurance is current.

For practitioners who must truthfully answer yes, or who have other credentialing flaws, does this mean that their applications will be rejected?

All applications require that *yes* answers be accompanied by detailed explanations and documentation of the specific circumstances. It's not possible to make a blanket statement regarding the chances of acceptance onto a managed care panel. Certainly the seriousness of the offense (if one was committed) will be a major determining factor, as will the needs of the overall network and the policies of the particular company. However, the current oversupply of clinicians in most areas probably will make acceptance onto the panel very difficult, all other things being equal. NCQA (2000), however, places no restriction on the ability of a managed care company to accept a professional with such a history. The Credentialing Committee, discussed later, has the responsibility of determining whether a professional's history of malpractice or other credentialing flaws is serious enough to prevent acceptance.

Managed Care Privileges

There are some applications that extend the loss-of-privileges question to include loss of participating-provider status from another managed care company. Some applications even go further and ask therapists to indicate—and provide a detailed explanation for—any voluntary resignations. This raises disturbing implications, addressed later in the sections on CVOs and the question of termination without cause.

Maintaining Our Own Confidentiality

The need to attest to the lack of health, mental health, or substance abuse conditions is also disturbing. What if there has been a record of substance abuse treatment? Managed care company policies with regard to accepting recovering professionals onto their networks, whether—and how—they monitor practitioners for continued sobriety, and what if any rights a recovering clinician has, are rarely made public.

With regards to a history of mental health treatment, some training programs and theoretical orientations require therapists to undergo their own therapy. The affidavit questions, however, seem to be more concerned with medication than psychotherapy. The implication is that a history of being prescribed psychotropic medications, or current use of them, is what is problematic and requires explanation.

Practitioners in recovery from substance abuse, who have been or are currently prescribed antidepressants or other psychotropic medication(s), or who have other concerns about revealing their health status, should consult an attorney knowledgeable about the Americans with Disabilities Act for guidance before answering the attestation questions or furnishing any information.

However clinicians may be advised to present themselves on applications, one thing is clear: It's better for professionals' confidentiality that we not use our own managed behavioral health benefits.

Outsourcing Credentialing

Due to the expense and amount of staff time involved, it is increasingly common for companies to contract with Credentialing Verification Organizations (CVOs). The CVO conducts the primary source verification and sends back a report for review by the credentialing committee.

The managed care company's use of a CVO means that the CVO gains access to a professional's personal and credentialing information.

The managed care company's use of a CVO means that the CVO gains access to a professional's personal and credentialing information. If a managed care company outsources their credentialing function to a CVO, the release of information the therapist is asked to sign is usually fearsomely inclusive, such as:

> I authorize The Credentialing Alliance (TCA) to inquire of any provider, hospital, graduate training program, university, internship/residency/fellowship program, professional association, state licensure board, professional liability carrier, personal reference, or any other individual or entity that can furnish information as to my clinical proficiency, personal character, physical health, emotional stability, professional ethics, or other matters pertaining to direct patient care. I authorize release of information by all individuals or entities contacted by TCA for purposes of credentialing.

> I further authorize TCA's release of information obtained to Healing Partners Behavioral Health (HPBH) pursuant to my application for participating-provider status.

> I hold TCA and HPBH harmless for actions performed in good faith during the credentialing process, in obtaining or releasing information about me for the purposes of evaluating my credentials.

Why must professionals be required to hold a CVO legally harmless? Their business is verifying information that can potentially cause harm to a therapist's ability to earn a living and maintain a good professional reputation. If they are not to be held responsible for errors, what is the incentive for the CVO to take all possible precautions to make sure that the information is correct?

Antitrust Concerns

The existence of CVOs creates the potential for companies to give provider-profiling information to the CVO, who can then pass it on to any other managed care company as part of that practitioner's file. United Healthcare, Oxford Health Plans, and Humana announced on June 15, 1999, their plan for a joint-venture physician credentialing project, through a CVO, Aperture (*Open Minds Advisor,* 1999). Such plans may save companies money, but have antitrust implications if competitors are shown to be colluding to prevent blackballed clinicians from joining panels to sell their services. The outcome of current antitrust litigation, such as *Holstein vs. Green Spring et al.* (1998), will presumably affect the way the CVOs operate in the future.

Know Your Rights

When applying for participating-provider status, find out if the managed care company is using a CVO, and get the CVO's address and phone number. Write a letter requesting a copy of your credentialing report. Include mention in the request that the right of practitioners to review their information and correct errors is part of NCQA's accreditation determination (NCQA 1998, 2000, CR 1.5–1.7). If there are any errors in the credentialing report, immediately notify both the CVO and the managed care company in writing, certified return receipt.

The right of practitioners to review their information and correct errors is part of NCQA's accreditation determination.

The Credentialing Committee

After credentialing, there is yet another step before an applicant can be upgraded to active participating network status. Every managed care company, even those which use CVOs, must have a *credentialing committee* that oversees credentialing decisions, operations, and procedures (NCQA, 2000, CR 2). The credentialing committee is made up of managed care company employees but also is required to include several participating professionals from a variety of disciplines. The managed care employees serving on the credentialing committee are typically managerial level network staff, with one or two managers from the clinical and/or QI departments, and a medical director. Smaller companies may have just one credentialing committee; the large MBHOs typically have regional credentialing committees reporting to a national committee.

If all an applicant's credentials are in order, the credentialing committee's approval is generally a formality.

If all an applicant's credentials are in order, the credentialing committee's approval is generally a formality. Because of the expense of credentialing, applications are only sent to those practitioners who are judged by the Network Development staff to be needed, as discussed in Chapter 2. The credentialing committee or another group of similar composition, including representation from panel clinicians, is also responsible for reviewing malpractice claims or other high-profile problems that may occur to practitioners who are already members of the panel, and deciding whether these practitioners can retain active network status. The credentialing committee is also in charge of recredentialing decisions.

Note that NCQA (2000, CR 3) imposes a 180-day time limit on information that has been primary source verified. If for some reason there is a logjam or other delay in approval by the credentialing committee, the managed care company is expected to re-contact the professional for another attestation, and is expected to perform a new primary source verification on all required information.

Recredentialing

In recredentialing, the professional's updated credentials, along with information on his or her performance as a member of the contracted network (the infamous provider profile), is sent to the credentialing committee for review and a decision about whether the therapist should continue as a member of the network.

It's no longer just a matter of sending in updated licenses, malpractice face sheets, and so on. Recredentialing is now a formal process that consists of most of the same steps, including primary source verification, as the original credentialing and NCQA (2000, CR 7) requires that it be performed every two years. Primary source verification is not performed again on items which won't have changed (i.e., one's degree), but the queries of the therapist's state licensure board, malpractice insurance carrier, the National Practitioner Data Bank, and all related primary source verifications will once again be undertaken.

In recredentialing, the professional's updated credentials, along with information on his or her performance as a member of the contracted network (*the infamous provider profile*), is sent to the credentialing committee for review and a decision about whether the therapist should continue as a member of the network. What sort of information is collected about practitioner performance?

Provider Profiling

Provider profiling refers to any method used to describe the members of the network. Although managed care companies do not deny engaging in *provider profiling,* each company considers its specific methods and profiling indicators to be proprietary information. Even on the inside, the case managers are not usually informed about the exact details of how network members are profiled and on what indicators.

There are, however, some measures common to all profiles, because the NCQA (2000, CR 9) specifies that the following information be taken into account as part of the recredentialing process:

- Member/patient complaints and satisfaction data.
- Clinical quality/outcomes data.

There are also other measures that are known to be part of professionals' profiles. The following were required for consideration in recredentialing by NCQA's 1998 standards, but were dropped in the 2000 version:

- Utilization data.
- Site visits.
- Treatment record reviews.

Other provider profiling measures include appointment accessibility (see Chapter 5), which can be determined via the member satisfaction surveys. Case managers' ratings contribute to the *"provider-profiling"* effort, and there's also an informal sort of *"provider profiling"* which goes on among managed care employees.

Satisfaction Ratings and Complaints

In addition to the measurement of client satisfaction, managed care companies are also required to keep careful track of client complaints and document their resolution (NCQA, 2000, RR 3.1). Patient/member satisfaction, complaints, and the resolution of complaints are important and relatively straightforward methods for organizations to use as a means of offering good customer service and responsiveness. But used as a part of the recredentialing process, the implication seems to be that too many complaints, or a low member satisfaction score, may cause the credentialing committee to decide to terminate that practitioner's contract.

Aside from the question of whether satisfaction and rate of complaints measures *quality* as opposed to customer service, this system risks setting in motion what Miller (1996) calls a *covert gag.* Instead of an official, contractual gag clause, Miller argues that the fear of customer complaints and dissatisfaction will cause therapists to *"put on a happy face"* and not inform clients about noncovered treatment options. This approach also does not seem to take into consideration that there might easily be therapeutic or clinical reasons for a patient's dissatisfaction, as anyone who has worked with borderline personality disorders well knows.

Clinical Quality/Outcomes Data

The newest trend in provider profiling is to use outcomes measures to answer the question, "Who is most effective at treating X diagnosis, and why? What are they doing that is so effective?"

The newest trend in *provider profiling* is to use outcomes measures to answer the question, "Who is most effective at treating X diagnosis, and why? What are they doing that is so effective?" Most companies use patient self-report measures, and are also integrating these into the utilization review process (see Chapter 8) and treatment guideline development process (see Chapter 7).

Utilization

A statistical analyst, typically employed by either the network or the quality department, gets data from paid claims that are broken down by practitioner, number of sessions, diagnosis, and other variables such as type of practice, type of reimbursement, discipline/license level, or geographical region. The average number of sessions per case per diagnosis may be a statistic in a therapist's profile, but this number means little except for purposes of comparsion with other practitioners. In other words, that Justa Therapist, PhD, has a sessions per case average of 17.3 for clients with Major Depression is relatively meaningless until it is compared with the averages of other professionals. If the national average for psychologists is 16.8 sessions, then Dr. Therapist's utilization isn't questionable. But if the average in her city for psychologists is 10.2, the company might begin to suspect a pattern of over-utilization. The common belief in the professional community is that the managed care companies use this data to feed referrals preferentially to whoever can accomplish the task in the fewest number of sessions. Managed care companies, on the other hand, argue that utilization data, when paired with outcomes data, can shed light as to the relative treatment effectiveness of various methods.

Under-utilization is also considered in addition to over-utilization. If terminating after too few sessions means that treatment was incomplete, then clients will most likely relapse and need additional treatment, which isn't cost-effective. And where there are case rate contracts (see Chapter 15), there is monitoring for under-utilization because of the inherent nature of this type of reimbursement arrangement.

Site visits and treatment record reviews are discussed in Chapter 4.

Case Manager Ratings

Case managers from at least three of the largest five companies indicated that the company's computer system was set up such that they could not complete their certifications or close a case without entering a rating. Case managers are typically asked to enter their opinion, using a Likert rating scale, on these issues:

> *The company's computer system was set up such that they could not complete their certifications or close a case without entering a rating.*

- The therapist's attitude toward managed care/receptiveness to case management.
- Timeliness of treatment reports.
- The practitioner's compliance with the company's rules and procedures.
- Was the treatment plan behavioral, goal-oriented, specific?
- Was the treatment plan targeted toward the presenting symptoms and diagnosis?
- Did the client improve?

Don't Want to Be Profiled?

Jerry Vaccaro, MD, medical director of PacifiCare Behavioral Health, and Kirk Griffith, PhD, of Magellan both indicated in interviews that accurate *provider profiling* depends on a reasonable sample size. So, relax! Receiving just a few clients per year doesn't allow a managed care company to make any meaningful conclusions about a therapist's performance. They do recognize that case mix, the fact that some clients have more severe problems than others with the same diagnosis, alters utilization, outcomes, and satisfaction data.

> *Receiving just a few clients per year doesn't allow a managed care company to make any meaningful conclusions about a therapist's performance.*

How many cases are needed to yield a valid profile? Dr. Griffith of Magellan stated that for their purposes, it would be a minimum of 10 to 20 cases per year, but cautioned that they are "still working on threshold sampling data and defining a minimum number of cases needed in order to be able to make conclusions about practice patterns." But is 10 cases enough? In a study of physician management of diabetes sponsored by the Agency for Healthcare Policy and Research, it was found that to have at least 80 percent reliability, each physician would have needed to treat 100 diabetic patients (Hofer et al., 1999).

It's an argument for staying small and staying solo. Large groups that receive a high volume of referrals are, naturally, going to be targeted for *provider-profiling* efforts.

Moving beyond the Paranoia of Provider Profiling

Provider-profiling practices raise uncomfortable suspicions. Managed care companies accuse professionals of not wanting to be accountable. Professionals accuse managed care companies of being solely motivated by profit and of secretly using data to steer referrals away from those whom the company perceives as a threat to their ability to control that profit.

I asked Drs. Griffith and Vaccaro how their respective companies are addressing practitioner fears associated with the process of *provider profiling*. Dr. Vaccaro described PacifiCare's approach to profiling as creating a dialogue: "For providers with enough volume, we profile them and send them feedback in letters which tell them 'in summary, here's how you're doing.' The letter compares the data to a norm of all other providers profiled and includes helpful hints." Does this allay fears or stimulate them? Dr. Vaccaro explained that "feedback from providers has been positive about the profiles. Of those surveyed, 85 percent said they liked them and 68 percent were positive even if they had been told they needed improvement. The fear is always *how are you going to use this against me* . . . we try to get people to see we're all in this together and are doing this to improve quality."

Dr. Griffith was likewise cognizant of practitioner fears in explaining Magellan's approach. "We want this to be a peer review, rather than an automated process. For each practitioner, there is an assigned professional provider review committee comprised of Magellan clinicians, and network provider representation among all disciplines. That group looks

at the data and makes determinations about utility. Then, if there is utility to the data, it gets pulled in to the recredentialing process."

A Simple Solution

Managed care does seem to be reaching out, but there needs to be still
greater efforts. Clearly, it's not a dialogue unless the profiled practitioner
has the right to give input, feedback, or ask questions—without fear of
the consequences of doing so. Therapists should be routinely invited to
take part, via teleconference, in their own recredentialing hearings when
their names come up before the committee. Instituting this right seems
to me to be the best and simplest solution to decrease the profound
suspicions engendered by *provider profiling*. After all, if there truly are
no skeletons to hide, why not open the closet door and let us see for
ourselves?

*Therapists should
be routinely
invited to take
part, via
teleconference, in
their own
recredentialing
hearings when
their names come
up before the
committee.*

Although the data from *provider profiling* can certainly be of use in the ongoing search for effective, quality treatments, it's imperative that managed
care companies—and NCQA—formally recognize that *provider profiling*
directly concerns the professional future of the therapists profiled. To
date, the only right offered to professionals is reactive, rather than proactive: the right of appeal once a recredentialing decision has been made
(NCQA, 1998, CR 10.2).

Informal Provider Profiling

> . . . There isn't a process in place to factor in the "sucking up" quotient, but
> it is a concern. . . . The best advice I have is that it's important for people to
> remember not to shoot the messenger. Remember you're talking to a human
> being, a peer. We're all trying to do our best. Don't take out your frustra-
> tions with the macro-economics [of managed care] on them if you want to
> maintain a relationship. I've had case managers in tears in my office be-
> cause of the way they were treated by practitioners.
> —Kirk Griffith, PhD, Senior Vice President of Clinical
> Network Management, Magellan Behavioral Health.

When you're looking to make a referral, it's easy to pass a name by. Isn't
that what everyone does? Case managers want to make their lives easy because the company piles it on.
> —Norman Hering, LMFT former case manager

*In the simplest,
most informal
form of provider
profiling
imaginable, case
managers talk to
each other.*

In the simplest, most informal form of *provider profiling* imaginable, case managers talk to each other.

> **Jill:** "Hey, Bob . . . know anything about Dr. John Q. Smith in Cleveland?"
>
> **Bob:** "Oh, don't use him if there's another psychiatrist close by . . . he never sends OTRs and he tells his clients to call to beg for re-certification."

Given Bob's bad experience, why would Jill, knowing nothing about Dr. Smith or the other network psychiatrists in Cleveland, then want to use Dr. Smith?

Termination without Cause

The most frightening implication of *provider profiling* is the possibility that one's status as a network participant might be terminated "without cause." Therapists stand to lose referrals and competitiveness in the marketplace. Patients lose their in-network benefits. Forever afterwards therapists will have to truthfully answer and explain that they were terminated from a managed care panel, even if there was no reason for the termination, such as loss of license or breach of contract. It will be a matter of public record, electronically verifiable.

Does No-Cause Termination Really Happen?

*Managed care
companies have
reasons for
wanting the ability
to terminate
contracted
professionals, such
as downsizing the
network, but these
reasons don't
permit a for-cause
termination.*

Managed care companies' contracts sometimes reserve the right to terminate professionals from the network without cause. As Kahn-Kothmann (1998) indicates, managed care companies have reasons for wanting the ability to terminate contracted professionals, such as downsizing the network, but these reasons don't permit a for-cause termination.

There are two distinct questions that must be answered when exploring the issue of no-cause terminations. The first addresses practitioners' fears regarding *provider profiling:* "Can it be proven that managed care companies systematically rid themselves of practitioners who they consider incompatible, or of those who strongly advocate for their patients, and/or of those who use more sessions than the companies would like to pay for?"

This first issue is about to be decided in court. The American Psychological Association sponsored a landmark case, *New Jersey Psychological*

Association (NJPA) vs. MCC Behavioral Care. Seven New Jersey psychologists challenged MCC Behavioral Care, a subsidiary of CIGNA (which has since changed its name to Cigna Behavioral Health), in 1996 after being terminated. The psychologists claimed that MCC labeled them "managed-care unfriendly" and gave them their pink slips as a result of having advocated for more sessions for their patients. The judge in the U.S. District Court of New Jersey ordered the case to proceed to trial over the objections of MCC (Rabasca, 1998).

The second question is a matter of policy, concerned with the balance of conflicting rights. On the one hand, maintaining a network is an expense for the managed care companies. However, managed care clearly exercises a great deal of influence over the ability of mental health professionals to sell their services in a free market. The balance of rights in health care delivery between professionals and managed care companies is an emerging legal question.

Describing recent cases, Kahn-Kothmann (1998) indicates that judicial opinion may be coming to rest on the side of practitioners and their patients. In *Harper vs. Healthsource New Hampshire, Inc.*, Paul Harper, a primary care physician, notified Healthsource of his concerns regarding patient records and for his medical integrity, was terminated from the HMO. The New Hampshire Supreme Court ultimately ruled that the public's interest is affected by an HMO's decision regarding the participating-provider status of one of its doctors, and that HMOs must therefore conduct themselves according to the legal principles of *fundamental fairness* and *good faith*.

Limbo-Listing and Accidental Removal from the Network

All of a sudden, out of the blue, a therapist or psychiatrist is told, "We're sorry, you're no longer an active part of the panel." It usually happens when the professional or a member of his or her office staff calls to ask why a certification didn't go through, or why a claim was denied. Sometimes a prospective client, requesting a particular therapist, or a client who has not been seen in a while, will be given this message when they call for precertification. This phenomenon is known as *limbo-listing;* practitioners lose their *active* status but are not openly terminated from the panel.

This phenomenon is known as limbo-listing; practitioners lose their active status but are not openly terminated from the panel.

Limbo-listed therapists' names can be programmed with computer codes that will withhold their names when an intake clinician or customer service rep does a search.

Limbo-listing is fairly easy for the managed care company, from a technical standpoint. Limbo-listed therapists' names can be programmed with computer codes that will withhold their names when an intake clinician or customer service rep does a search, thus effectively blocking the therapist from receiving referrals.

Think you've been limbo-listed? Calling Provider Relations is probably not the best course of action. The rep who answers the line might not be able to be of much help, either because the information is not available to someone at such a low level, or because there are instructions not to reveal it. Instead, take the following steps:

1. Follow up *immediately* on *anything* that looks like removal from the panel which was done without a clear letter of intent to do so from the managed care company.

2. Speak to Claims or Customer Service first, if the reason for the suspicion about limbo-listing or a network-status problem is due to a claim paid out-of-network. Proceed to Provider Relations only if the Claims/Customer Service employee cannot fix the problem.

3. Once on the phone with a Provider Relations employee, ask only one thing: "What is my current network status?" Don't argue with anything the Provider Relations rep says. Don't ask about rankings or listings on search programs. The rep is not going to have, or is not going to be allowed to reveal, that information.

4. Request that the managed care company send immediate written confirmation of your active participating-provider status. It's a reasonable, although not common, request. Politely but firmly ask to speak to a supervisor if the request is refused or the rep tries to argue.

5. Persist. If the written confirmation never arrives, keep calling back. Ask to speak to a supervisor, then go as high as need be beyond the immediate supervisor, until the written confirmation arrives.

6. Discreet, casual references to the NCQA, the state Department of Insurance, U.S. Senators, or Congressional Representatives may be helpful. Just be sure to stay nice; don't threaten.

7. Make numerous copies of the letter; send one attached to each batch of claims.

Limbo-listing doesn't get around NCQA's requirement that the MBHO or its delegate recredential each professional every two years, but an "accidental" removal from the network does. Sometimes accidental removal truly is an accident and not some sort of conspiracy. Network departments, which have thousands of names to track, do make mistakes. A former Network Development Manager who was interviewed, commented that "the provider database contained a lot of errors." She continued, "Decisions were made, often appearing arbitrary, that would inactivate a provider from the database. It was not clear why the decision was made, but often the clinician was not informed of the change in his or her status." Mergers and acquisitions play havoc as well (see Chapter 4).

Sometimes accidental removal truly is an accident and not some sort of conspiracy.

Then there's the problem with documentation being lost during the recredentialing process or when making changes which require notifying the managed care company. Following up is imperative with recredentialing information or changes (Table 3.1).

One of the most effective ways managed care organizations trim the network is to lose documentation (intentionally or not), and then invoke the "Provider must promptly notify Ultra-Care Behavioral Health of license renewal" contract clause, terminating the therapist for breach. On appeal, a certified return receipt card might be the key to victory. Keep it in a file with network contracts and other managed care company information.

Following up is imperative with recredentialing information or changes.

If your response is, "That's just too much bother, let them do what they want. I never get that many referrals anyway," remember that it's no longer just about participating in the network of one particular company. Even if a therapist no longer has any interest in being on a company's panel, an alleged breach of contract goes on a professional's permanent records and may effectively deter other managed care companies from

Table 3.1
Survival Tips for "Ordinary Notifications"

- Keep records of the date and nature of each contact with a Provider Relations representative, including the name of the person and their extension.
- Promptly send in copies of license and malpractice renewals certified return receipt requested. That green return receipt card is proof of having notified the managed care company if they end up losing the information.
- Promptly notify the company of any change in Tax ID, name, address, or telephone number in writing, certified return receipt requested.
- Follow up with Provider Relations 4 to 6 weeks after the return receipt of any correspondence or updates, to verify that the requested information or changes were documented. Make a record of the time and date of the call, the name of the employee, and the content of the conversation.

accepting his or her future applications. Fighting to stay on a managed care network might not be worth the hassle, but what about fighting to retain a professional good name?

Guerrilla Tactics in the Fight against "Limbo-Listing" or Accidental Removal

If possible, get a complete participating-provider list from the managed care company every 6 to 12 months and check for the presence of your name. This isn't easy, but there are two strategies that are likely to work, especially with the very large carve-out managed behavioral care companies.

Callers who are ineligible, but who say, "I just need to know who's on the directory before I can make a decision about whether to go with this plan" shouldn't have any problem.

1. *The prospective insured approach:* Call the managed care company (or have a friend or family member do it). Explain to the customer service rep that you are considering an insurance plan which uses this managed care company for the mental health/substance abuse benefit. Callers who are ineligible, but who say, "I just need to know who's on the directory before I can make a decision about whether to go with this plan" shouldn't have any problem. Insist on obtaining a complete list of therapists matching your credentials within 10 miles of your office zip code.

2. *The referring therapist approach:* Find a colleague of the opposite gender or a different discipline or specialty, located within 10 miles of your office's zip code, who has similar concerns. Each of you should call the managed care company separately and request a complete list of practitioners of your partner's discipline, gender, or specialty. Use the explanation that it is important for you to have this information on hand for clients who need referrals. Be sure to state clearly that you understand that the network might change, and that the client always must call to verify network status and precertify. Then, exchange lists.

Caught in the Crossfire: Patients Currently in Therapy

Regardless of the cause of network status difficulties, the primary concern must always be for the welfare of patients currently receiving services.

Clients have a fundamental right to uninterrupted, benefit-covered treatment until the current episode of care is completed. Managed care companies generally honor this right, although often the therapist must act as an advocate for patients in order to get it to happen.

Acting as Client Advocate

The most frequent reason therapists must act as advocates for their clients is simply because the large carve-out managed behavioral care companies are disorganized. The seemingly endless series of mergers has done its share to account for the disorganization, but any large corporate system is similar. One division or department acts independently of the others, without recognition of the consequences for other parts of the system. Even with all our amazing technology, things still drop through the cracks.

The case manager usually has no power to re-instate a therapist's network status, but can use the *ad-hoc* technique (see Chapter 2) to make sure that the client's claims are paid and the certification process goes (*relatively*) smoothly. When talking to the case manager, keep the focus on the client and his or her needs.

Be wary of "transitional" sessions. It generally is fairly easy to get the managed care company to authorize continued in-network benefit reimbursement until the end of the treatment episode. Occasionally, though, a very profit-driven managed care company will say something like, "We'll give the client 5 more sessions to make the decision whether to continue to see you and use out-of-network benefits/pay out-of-pocket or to transfer to a participating provider."

Transitional sessions are not acceptable, but don't say that to the case manager, or show anger. This is a clinician with no power (sound familiar?) who is probably cringing inside. If this is the answer, thank the case manager for his or her advocacy on behalf of the client, take the 4 or 6 sessions, and plan the next move.

Some states are considering patient-protection laws to the effect that patients who begin treatment with a plan specialist must have their in-network reimbursement guaranteed for a certain length of time, or until the end of the treatment episode, even if the specialist is dropped from the network. Write to the state Department of Insurance to file a complaint and/or inquire about what protections the state offers.

Clients have a fundamental right to uninterrupted, benefit-covered treatment until the current episode of care is completed.

When talking to the case manager, keep the focus on the client and his or her needs.

Another alternative is to strike at the managed care company just where they fear it most; by complaining—in writing—to the entity that has awarded them the contract.

Another alternative is to strike at the managed care company just where they fear it most; by complaining—in writing—to the entity that has awarded them the contract. Explain to the client the option of writing to Human Resources at his or her employer, or the benefit administrator of his or her health plan, letting these influential individuals know of the lack of continuity of care and nonexistent commitment to quality demonstrated by the managed care company. If the client doesn't mind public exposure, consider using the media and/or appealing to legislators and congressional representatives. Managed care companies generally would rather give in than get more negative PR; these days, they get plenty of that.

Resignation doesn't carry the same ethical obligations to the client on the part of the managed care company. Voluntarily resigning in the middle of treatment with a patient who is using his or her in-network benefits places the burden of working out financial arrangements squarely on the shoulders of the therapist. The trick, for therapists planning to resign but waiting to finish out a client's therapy, is to call the managed care company, and request a hold-all-referrals status.

Reasons managed care companies will grant temporary inactive status:

1. Vacations.
2. A full practice.
3. Medical illness.

4

The Managed Care Contract

Signing Your Life Away: The Participating-Provider Contract

Disclaimer: This section should in no way be considered a substitute for reading the actual managed care contract(s). Each company's contract will be slightly different in language and specific features. Seek advice from a knowledgeable lawyer for questions about participating-provider contracts. Although it's usually not possible to negotiate or change the terms of managed care company contracts, knowledge of contract specifications is the only way to make an informed decision about whether signing the contract/staying on the panel is in your best interests.

The most critical thing to keep in mind is that these contracts are drafted by highly paid lawyers working for the managed care company, and naturally, the terms will be favorable to the company—not to practitioners. An attorney to represent your interests is an important resource.

Some of the most important features of a participating-provider contract are the miscellaneous provisions. Most contracts begin with a series of definitions. Although reading these may be the world's new miracle cure for insomnia, it's probably a good idea. The level of detail of this section varies considerably from one company to another, but don't let the label "miscellaneous" mislead you into thinking it's not important.

Independent Contractor. All contracts contain a statement to the effect that the relationship of the private practitioner to the managed care company is that of an independent contractor, not an employee. It seems basically innocuous and obvious, although the implications are anything but. Independent contractors, unlike employees who can join a union, are not legally able to bargain collectively for better working conditions

Although it's usually not possible to negotiate or change the terms of managed care company contracts, knowledge of contract specifications is the only way to make an informed decision about whether signing the contract/ staying on the panel is in your best interests.

or fees. If they should try, they would be considered as being in collusion to fix or restrain trade—a federal antitrust violation.

Nonexclusivity.   Following the statement about being an independent contractor, there is usually language to the effect that nothing in the contract prohibits the professional from signing similar contracts with other managed care or insurance companies. They're not including this clause out of generosity. Managed care companies include such a statement as one piece of evidence that participating therapists are independent contractors rather than employees, by the standards of the Internal Revenue Service who defines what constitutes an "independent contractor" versus an "employee."

Indemnify/Hold Harmless.   Indemnification clauses are often part of managed care contracts and mean that if the company is named in a lawsuit, the therapist pays for the defense. Some indemnification clauses are now two-way; the therapist agrees not to hold the managed care company liable for any reason, but the managed care company also agrees not to hold the therapist liable (Zieman, 1998).

Malpractice insurance policies typically don't pay for therapists' contractual indemnification obligations to the managed care company, unless the company has previously been specifically endorsed on the policy.

It's the "one-way" indemnification clause, where the therapist agrees to protect the managed care company, but not the other way around, that can be dangerous. Bernstein (1998) reminds professionals that malpractice insurance policies typically don't pay for therapists' contractual indemnification obligations to the managed care company, unless the company has previously been specifically endorsed on the policy. Usually, there is an additional fee for endorsing a managed care company; however, it might be the best and only protection for therapists whose managed care contract(s) include a "one-way" indemnification clause. Malpractice carriers can offer more specific advice about the costs and advisability of taking this step.

Noncompete Clause.   It's not at all the same thing as nonexclusivity. Noncompete clauses prohibit the participating professional from soliciting away the businesses contracted with the managed care organization. This doesn't really apply to therapists in solo practice, but it is an issue for large groups, IPAs, or integrated delivery systems, who may have signed participating-provider contracts with the managed care organizations, while at the same time competing with them in the direct contracting and EAP market.

Professional Liability or Malpractice Insurance. The company expects professionals to maintain a certain minimum level of insurance coverage (usually more for MDs than for the other disciplines). These paragraphs place responsibility on the professional to furnish the managed care company with proof of insurance and renewals as they occur. Then there's typically a statement indicating that if there is a claim, cancellation, or significant change in malpractice insurance status, the clinician must notify the managed care company, usually within a specified amount of time.

Obligation to Report. This section may also be known as *Notice of Actions* or *Notice Obligations.* Whatever they call it, it's not referring to the mandatory reporting of child/elder abuse, or Tarasoff situations, or anything clinical. It has to do with things a contracted clinician must report to the managed care company within a certain time frame specified by the contract, usually 2 to 5 business days. Some situations, such as licensure and malpractice insurance expiration and renewal, happen to everyone and copies of the renewed materials must be sent to the company. Other contractual obligations happen only in the event of more unusual circumstances, such as suspension or loss of license. The typical situations in which managed care companies contractually require immediate notice from professionals are:

If there is a claim, cancellation, or significant change in malpractice insurance status, the clinician must notify the managed care company, usually within a specified amount of time.

- Ordinary changes: license/malpractice insurance renewal, change of name, address, phone number, legal status change (i.e., a group incorporates or disbands), or tax ID change.
- Any malpractice action filed. (Contracts generally stipulate that the reporting to the managed care company must be made when the suit is filed, not upon conviction or acquittal.)
- Loss, restriction, suspension, or sanction against professional license or DEA certificate.
- Investigation, disciplinary hearings, sanction, or proceedings by professional organizations, Medicare, Medicaid, CHAMPUS, and/or state licensure boards for either professional misconduct or billing fraud.
- Loss of hospital privileges.
- Civil or criminal actions filed (filing, not conviction).
- Loss, reduction of, or cancellation of malpractice insurance (as described above).

*Contracts
generally also
include a "not
otherwise
specified" clause
that states the
professional must
notify the
managed care
company
immediately upon
any other
situation or
change that might
affect the ability
to deliver services
as contracted.*

Reporting Obligations, NOS.   Contracts generally also include a "not otherwise specified" clause that states the professional must notify the managed care company immediately upon any other situation or change that might affect the ability to deliver services as contracted. For instance, if you will be traveling abroad for 6 months, undergoing intensive chemotherapy, or simply have a full practice, let the managed care company know that you will not be available for referrals. Provider Relations generally will accept a phone call as sufficient notice, and will inactivate a therapist's name until he or she calls in again and indicates once more being ready to receive referrals. In such situations, even if an end date to the blackout period was given at the time of the original call, it's still a good idea to call back to reactivate network status.

Advertising.   Not all contracts include this provision. It gives permission to the managed care company to list the therapist's name in whatever advertising or marketing measures they may use, most commonly a printed directory. Even though managed behavioral carve-outs rarely print directories, the contract reserves their right to do so.

Advertising clauses may also ban the therapist from using the managed care company's logo/name and the logos/names of its customers in the therapist's or group practice's marketing materials. However, it does not generally preclude therapists stating on practice profiles that they are an *independent contractor, participating provider, network provider,* or *independent contracted therapist* for XYZ Behavioral Healthcare.

Quality Improvement Initiatives.   Older contracts typically don't include this section, which requires professionals to participate in any and all Quality Improvement, outcomes measurement, or data-collection programs initiated by the company. You guessed it: such a contract clause is required by NCQA for managed care companies to achieve accreditation (NCQA, 2000, QI 3.1.1 & QI 3.2.1).

Mandatory Arbitration.   Contracts may specify that any disputes which cannot be directly resolved between the professional and the managed care company must be arbitrated. If arbitration is mandated, typically the therapist is required to accept the independent arbitrator's decision as final and binding, and must agree not to take the matter to court. The contract may then spell out the conditions and procedures for the arbitration.

What Can Be Disclosed?

Proprietary Information and Materials. Also referred to as a *Nondisclosure* clause, the managed care company forbids the practitioner to reveal any and all information about its fees, policies, procedures, forms, medical necessity criteria, and so on. It differs from a *gag clause* only in who is the recipient of the information. *Gag clauses* refer to disclosures to patients; nondisclosure clauses are aimed at other professionals, other managed care companies, and the general public. Companies generally consider nondisclosure to be one of a professional's ongoing responsibilities even after the termination of the contract. Managed care companies argue that this information is "proprietary" and could cause them to lose competitive advantage if revealed.

And that, says antitrust attorney Joseph Sahid, is the legal purpose of these clauses. If a therapist went to one company and cited specifics of how other companies work (or what they pay), in an attempt to get more money, less paperwork, or other advantages, the therapist could be in legal trouble. Nor can we professionals collectively bargain for better fees. However, says Sahid, the managed care companies word the nondisclosure clauses such that they are "overly broad and therefore unenforceable. . . . Courts generally support contractual prohibitions only if they are reasonable in scope." Sahid's opinion is that the proprietary information clauses in managed care contracts probably look a lot scarier than they really are. "The managed care companies keep these clauses broad as a threat."

Can we talk about fees? Sahid explains that as long as sharing contract-specific information is not done in an attempt to convince colleagues to act in accordance with an agenda which might be construed as price-fixing or antitrust in nature (such as boycotting a particular managed care company whose fees are too low), the disclosure is probably not going to place a therapist in jeopardy.

But when in doubt, play it safe: consult an attorney, or do not reveal. No one wants to become the next test case. Attorney and social work professor Bart Bernstein, coauthor of *The Portable Lawyer for Mental Health Professionals* (John Wiley, 1999), stated in an interview, "We have to keep in mind that this whole field, legally, is very new. From a judicial standpoint, there is no body of case law yet."

Also referred to as a Nondisclosure clause, the managed care company forbids the practitioner to reveal any and all information about its fees, policies, procedures, forms, medical necessity criteria, and so on.

When in doubt, play it safe: consult an attorney, or do not reveal.

A gag clause in a managed care company contract is any restriction regarding what the therapist can tell the patient about the noncovered— or more expensive— treatment options or the behind-the-scenes financial incentives that favor certain treatments, or shorter therapy. These clauses are now outlawed in a number of states and by the NCQA, JCAHO, and other accreditation entities.

The Infamous *Gag Rule.*   A *gag clause* in a managed care company contract is any restriction regarding what the therapist can tell the patient about the noncovered—or more expensive—treatment options or the behind-the-scenes financial incentives that favor certain treatments, or shorter therapy. These clauses are now outlawed in a number of states and by the NCQA, JCAHO, and other accreditation entities.

Dig out your contract and check the date it was signed. If the contract date is 1998 or before, it may contain a gag clause. If the gag clause is present, follow the contract procedures for proposing an amendment. Write a letter requesting the elimination of the gag clause, mentioning in writing that per NCQA Standard QI 3.1.3 (NCQA, 2000) for accreditation of managed behavioral healthcare organizations, "the organization allows open practitioner-patient communication." Have a lawyer review the letter, and copy it to the state Department of Insurance if your state has banned gag rules. Response by the managed care company should be slow but favorable; however, there's always the option of copying the letter to NCQA if they decide to stonewall.

Audits

Contracts reserve the right to audit records, either as part of a site visit to the professional's office, or by requesting that complete treatment records be sent to the managed care company—at the practitioner's expense, of course. NCQA standards mandate that managed behavioral care companies conduct at least one site visit and one treatment record review of "high volume" professionals (NCQA, 2000, CR 6). For solo practitioners, the definition of "high volume" is up to the managed care companies; however, NCQA does require a site visit/treatment record review for all locations of all group practices on the panel.

What happens during a site visit? It's unquestionably an expense for the therapist. The managed care company is supposed to give "reasonable" notice of their intent to visit ("reasonable" is not always spelled out in the contract!). In practice, this should be at least 3 to 4 weeks' notice. Site visitors mean that clients cannot be scheduled during the visit, due to confidentiality. Although the walk-through of the office will take less than an hour from start to finish, the loss of income includes whatever time the practitioner has spent in preparation.

Pretend It's Your Mother-in-Law Paying a Visit.   Site visitors are looking to see if maximum confidentiality is ensured through the physical layout and arrangements in the office. Table 4.1 lists ways to improve confidentiality.

Additionally, site visitors inspect offices with an eye toward physical safety of clients and professional appearance. With regard to safety, this means things like fire alarms/smoke detectors, fire extinguishers, clearly marked exits, sprinkler systems, adequate ventilation, and so on. *Professional appearance* certainly is a relative term, but if the office is clean, the furniture is intact, the magazine rack isn't filled with pornography, and the stereo isn't blasting heavy metal music, it's probably OK. And, although I consider this shamefully discriminatory to our four-legged friends, who can be as therapeutic as we are, pets are a no-no, because some people are allergic (fish are OK, though).

Site visitors will also look to see if the office is in reasonable proximity to public transportation (2–3 blocks at most, if the area has public transportation). They will prefer free and plentiful off-street parking. They will note the cleanliness and privacy of the restrooms. And they will check to see what kinds of accommodations exist in the office and in the building for people with disabilities (ramps, elevators, automatic doors, etc.).

Kirk Griffith, PhD, senior vice president at Clinical Network Management, Magellan Behavioral Health, offered an additional tip on getting

Site visitors are looking to see if maximum confidentiality is ensured through the physical layout and arrangements in the office.

Table 4.1
Does Your Office Promote Confidentiality?

- Are there separate entrances and exits?
- Are there separate waiting rooms (not generally mandatory, but a nice plus)?
- Do the consulting rooms/therapist offices ensure privacy (i.e., soundproofing adequate such that clients in the waiting room and office staff cannot overhear)?
- Are the files kept locked at all times?
- Where is the filing cabinet located? Is it in an area that can be locked?
- Are computers password-protected?
- Are communication devices such as copiers, answering machines, and fax machines kept secure (i.e., where patients or other unauthorized individuals cannot see/hear the output)?
- How has the practitioner trained the office staff in regards to maintaining confidentiality? Are there signed confidentiality agreements? Written office confidentiality policies?
- How is confidentiality maintained from janitorial/housekeeping staff?
- Does the clinician's release of information form comply with all local, state, and managed care company/ NCQA standards?

ready for site visits. "We want to see that providers have a structured orientation to maintaining patient's rights. Providers should have written formal procedures for this. Even solo practitioners should have something in writing." Specifically, he suggested, post members' rights in a prominent location.

Don't panic! An office isn't expected to be perfect—site visitors usually have a checklist and the expectation is that the office will score yes to a certain percentage of the items. They also rarely kick people out of the network on the spot due to the results of a site visit. Reviewers who notice something serious are instructed to counsel the clinician about it at the time of the visit and make a corrective plan with a follow-up visit.

They also rarely kick people out of the network on the spot due to the results of a site visit.

Home Offices. The general rule with a home office is that the same expectations apply as with any other office. It's considered mandatory that there be a separate entrance/exit from the rest of the house, and that the office has restricted access to and from the living quarters. So, therapists whose living room is also their waiting room should consider resigning if the managed care company announces a site visit! Those working from home must be able to demonstrate that the room(s) in which therapy takes place, and where the phone, fax, computer, copier, answering machine, and records are stored, are private and not accessible to the rest of the family, neighbors, pets, and so on.

Treatment Record Audits. This might be one of the few advantages that NCQA offers the professional community—standardization of expectations. It's easier to be accountable to one system than to go crazy trying to meet the slightly-differing expectations of each of the ten different companies with which one might be contracted. NCQA-compliant standards for documentation can be found in any recently-revised (1998 or later) provider manual from a major managed behavioral care organization.

NCQA (1998, 2000) requires that 24 elements be present in a clinical treatment record (Table 4.2). For at least part of a record review, giving the auditors a copy of a blank patient record form (on paper or computer disk) may be sufficient. The reviewers are going to look for the presence of fields for the necessary information, rather than for the information itself. For the rest, a blinded record is the next best solution, and this should be as close as an auditor should come to a "live" chart.

The reviewers are going to look for the presence of fields for the necessary information, rather than for the information itself.

Financial Audits. Site reviewers from a managed care company will ask to look at financial documentation, to make sure all is in compliance

Table 4.2
How Would Your Treatment Records Fare in an Audit?

1. *Administrative elements:*

   - Patient name/ID on *every* page of the record.
   - Patient intake data (home and work/school address and phone, emergency contact info, marital status, and informed consent forms).
   - Each entry is signed off with credentials included.
   - Entries must be dated.
   - Legible.

2. *Psychosocial/Assessment Data:*

   - Presenting problem(s) described, including the biopsychosocial factors affecting the presenting problem(s).
   - Previous treatment (medical and psychiatric) information including dates, who/where, any consultation with former providers or review of previous treatment records, family medical/psychiatric history, lab tests, other sources of information such as previous testing, collateral contacts, and so on.
   - Complete alcohol/drug evaluation. In addition to illicit drugs, the assessment should include over-the-counter and prescription drugs as well as nicotine. Past as well as present use, past treatment, consequences of use, and relevant family history (for all clients over age 12).
   - Documented mental status evaluation.
   - *DSM-IV* diagnosis, all axes. The reviewer will expect diagnosis to follow from the symptoms/problems reported or observed in the mental status evaluation, presenting issues, and history.

3. *Medical Information:*

   - Description of medical conditions included in the record.
   - Medications, dosages, and dates of prescription/refill(s) noted.
   - Allergies and any side effects to medication(s).
   - If no known allergies, document that this was asked.

4. *Risk Factors/Risk Management:*

   - Suicidal/homicidal ideation, imminent risk of harm to self/others, and the presence/absence of other risk factors are documented, along with safety precautions if risk is present.
   - If clients decompensate (i.e., suicidal, unable to perform ADLs), interventions are made and documented which refer client to a higher level of care until stable again.

5. *If Patient Is a Child or Adolescent:*

   - Biopsychosocial, educational, and developmental history including any prenatal/perinatal factors of importance (or documentation of the absence of such factors).

(continued)

Table 4.2 (Continued)

6. *Progress Notes and Treatment Plan:*

- Goals consistent with diagnoses and are written in behavioral, measurable, and specific format including estimated length of treatment.
- Documented interventions follow from and are consistent with the goals listed on the treatment plan.
- Documentation of client understanding and consent to specific treatment plan, and/or consent for medication, should be present.
- Progress notes should include assessment of client strengths/obstacles to achievement of goals as listed on treatment plan. Modifications to treatment plan are documented.
- Use of community resources and preventive services, as appropriate.
- Documentation of consultation and coordination with other professionals involved with client (i.e., including but not limited to primary care MD).

7. *Discharge:*

- Discharge/relapse prevention plan, including dates of follow-up appointments or contacts.

Adapted from NCQA (1998, 2000), *Guidelines for Treatment Record Review,* © NCQA. Used with permission.

with the company's policies. Most contracts do reserve the right to examine financial accounts for their beneficiaries. They're looking to:

1. Make sure no copayments were waived (see Chapter 14).
2. Make sure the patient has not been balance-billed.
3. Make sure that there is informed consent on the patient's part for payment of noncovered services.
4. Determine that there is no systematic pattern of charging more to insurance patients than to others (see Chapter 14).

What They Do and Don't Have a Right to Inspect. I can't think of any situation in which a managed care auditor would have the right to look at clinical records from any client who is not a covered beneficiary. There are horror stories floating about that sometimes auditors will request other records "for purposes of comparison." In the unlikely event of this occurring, refuse the request and report the auditor in writing to the managed care company, with a copy of the complaint to the state Insurance Department and NCQA. The letter should state your willingness to cooperate with any audit process that does not violate other patients' confidentiality.

However, financial data is different. As a general rule, aggregate information (i.e., income summary reports, accounts receivable reports)

> *I can't think of any situation in which a managed care auditor would have the right to look at clinical records from any client who is not a covered beneficiary.*

and/or blinded individual client financial records may be considered "fair game" for the managed care company's inspection during an audit. Check with an attorney if there are any questions regarding what an auditor does/does not have a right to examine.

Changing the Contract and/or Getting Out

Contract Amendment Process

Contracts are either for a fixed term, or are self-perpetuating, which means that the contract will be automatically renewed when the term concludes. If there were no clause for automatic renewal, then the managed care company would be forced to send out new contracts at the end of each term. Needless to say, this would be an expensive and staff intensive process, so all managed care companies include clauses in their contracts that allow for the contract to be automatically renewed at the end of the term.

All managed care companies include clauses in their contracts that allow for the contract to be automatically renewed at the end of the term.

So how are changes (amendments) made to the contracts? Therapists tend to assume that once they've signed a managed care contract, the company can issue fee reductions or other mandates from on high and there is nothing they can do about it except resign. Wrong. There is always a statement in the reams of fine print that addresses the issue of making amendments.

Proposing Changes.   It's not just the managed care company that can make changes. Professionals can too; at least in theory. Typically the contract will state that the clinician must notify the managed care company in writing, and obtain consent in writing, in order for the change to be considered legally binding and part of the ongoing contract. The difficulty will be in obtaining the managed care company's written consent.

Responding to Changes Proposed by the Company.   There's a seemingly harmless little paragraph that gives therapists the contractual right to fight fee reductions or other changes. It says that when the company announces changes, practitioners have a certain window of time (usually 30 days) to file objections in writing. Not responding within the time frame is interpreted to mean acceptance of the change, which then officially goes into effect, modifying the contract. If there is an objection, this paragraph generally elaborates the process of negotiation

When the company announces changes, practitioners have a certain window of time (usually 30 days) to file objections in writing.

to be undertaken by the company and the professional (see Chapter 14 for advice on using this strategy to fight fee reductions).

Resignation

Resignations MUST be in writing, no exceptions. Contracts typically require therapists to give at least 30 days' written notice of intent to resign.

Would that it were as easy as saying "Take this job and shove it!" Unfortunately, it's not. Resignations MUST be in writing, no exceptions. Contracts typically require therapists to give at least 30 days' written notice of intent to resign. Check the contract; some companies actually require longer notice periods of up to 45 or 60 days. Don't worry; the notice period does not require therapists to take new referrals during that time. What it does do is permit a window of opportunity to make other arrangements for existing clients, should they wish transfer to a network participant. Naturally, send the resignation letter certified return receipt or via any other method which allows for proof of delivery.

Breach of Contract and Termination.   The contract usually includes a remedy if either party believes the other to be in breach of the agreement. Most commonly, the party believing that there has been a breach must notify the other side in writing, allowing a certain number of days for the breach to be fixed. If the problem is corrected to the satisfaction of both sides, the contract remains in force; otherwise, it is terminated after the specified number of days. These contract clauses generally also specify other conditions of for-cause termination and the practitioner's right to appeal such termination. There may also to be a statement to the effect that the company reserves the right to alter its network composition and terminate the practitioner without cause (see Chapter 3).

Like a nasty divorce, you're never completely rid of them. Certain of the managed care contractual terms remain binding on professionals even after the contract has ended, and regardless of which party initiated the dissolution of the contractual relationship. These obligations generally include:

- Maintaining confidentiality (of course).
- Continuing treatment of any and all patients covered by that managed care company until clinically appropriate arrangements are made.
- Maintaining records.
- Adhering to financial contract obligations for services rendered when the therapist was still under contract.

- Any contract terms specifying nondisclosure of proprietary information and/or use of copyrighted forms.

Becoming Part of an Inheritance: Mergers and Acquisitions

"But I never signed a contract with this company!" Managed care employees hear this on an almost daily basis from someone or other in the network. The rampant mergers and acquisitions over the past decade are almost entirely responsible for situations in which therapists find themselves members of networks for which they have not signed contracts. The answer is usually found buried among the legalese of a participating-provider contract which was signed. Somewhere, often found in a section called *Assignment,* is a statement worded something like this:

> GenRUs Behavioral Health, Inc., may assign this contractual agreement to a successor entity in conjunction with a merger or acquisition involving GBH or a parent corporation.

Managed care companies which buy other companies are also buying those companies' networks. Contracted therapists are a commodity, no different from the computer infrastructure used by the service centers. And as a commodity, networks are bought and sold on the open market. Generally speaking, whatever the new corporate entity wishes to do with the network(s) when everything is integrated is up to them.

What happens to practitioners when managed care companies merge or acquire each other? Participating-provider contracts typically remain in force, with the terms unchanged, until officially altered or replaced with a contract redesigned by the new (merged) company, under its new corporate identity.

Integrating Giants

In the largest merger of managed behavioral health carve-out organizations in the short history of managed care, Magellan Health Services, at that time co-owner of the Charter psychiatric hospital chain and Green Spring Health Services, bought Human Affairs International (HAI) at the end of 1997, and Merit Behavioral Care (MBC) in early 1998. How

The rampant mergers and acquisitions over the past decade are almost entirely responsible for situations in which therapists find themselves members of networks for which they have not signed contracts.

Managed care companies which buy other companies are also buying those companies' networks.

does integration of managed behavioral care companies play out? Over a period of several years. Kirk Griffith, PhD, Senior Vice President of Clinical Network Management at Magellan, shared his thoughts on Magellan's integration efforts: "Until we move providers over to Magellan contracts, we have to abide by terms of their original contracts with the legacy companies." Sometimes, said Dr. Griffith, new contracts are presented when the individual professional comes up for recredentialing. But the recredentialing cycle is apparently not the only, or even the most major, factor. "You have to take into account government and state regulations, legal issues, and customer contract specifications."

"Customer contract specifications" refers to the fact that the managed care company's service contracts with each employer, union, insurance company, state, or local government vary widely in their nature and their specifications, determined by the sales/RFP process. It's apparently not as simple as just saying, "OK guys, we're now Magellan, and we're now going to do things Magellan's way." Dr. Griffith confirmed this, stating, "We have to get permission from customers to make changes."

Why does it take several years to fully integrate? This is just an overview of some of what must occur when managed care companies merge:

- Centralize and unify national and regional management.
- Centralize and unify employee/human resources issues.
- Develop new policies, procedures, documentation, and so on, for the merged company.
- Computer operating system conversions.
- Develop participating-provider contracts for the new company.
- Combine participating-provider networks.
- Continue the recredentialing cycle.
- Equalize fees for the merged companies for the same CPT/license in the same geographic area.
- Consolidate duplicate systems (i.e., claims payment centers).
- Assure existing customers of the merged companies that the new entity will continue to provide quality, satisfactory services.
- Comply with legal and regulatory requirements in each state where the merged company operates.
- Bid on new business as a merged entity and implement the new accounts.

After this quick glimpse into the corporate complexities involved in the integration of managed behavioral care organizations, and the length of time the process takes from start to finish, imagine the chaos if there is a new merger or acquisition every year.

Other Consequences of the Assignment Clause

Assignment is a one-way street. Not to be confused with the billing term *accepting assignment* (see Chapter 14), the *Assignment* clause is often used to forbid the transferring of the contract from one therapist to another. People do want to do that, occasionally, especially in instances where practices are sold. Unlike buying a managed care company, where the network is included, buying a practice does not confer the seller's participating-provider status on the purchaser.

Additions to Groups

Just like buying a practice, joining a group practice that has a group contract with the managed care company does not automatically convey participating-provider status. There is usually a page of the contract that lists the members of the group. New group members needing to be added must still go through the individual credentialing process, and must obtain the managed care company's approval to be added to the contract. It can be a difficult and time-consuming process to add new group members in full markets.

No Supervision

Assignment clauses also specify that all work with patients is to be done by the therapist who signed the contract. Managed care companies almost never reimburse for services provided by another professional who is under the supervision of the contracted therapist.

Buying a practice does not confer the seller's participating-provider status on the purchaser.

Joining a group practice that has a group contract with the managed care company does not automatically convey participating-provider status.

5

Getting Referrals and Getting Them Scheduled

Sarah, who lives in a Chicago suburb, called the number on her insurance card to get a referral to see a therapist for her anxiety. After a telephone assessment with a GBH counselor, Rita, Sarah indicated a preference for a female therapist. Rita gave her 3 names of female therapists, all very close to her home, and explained Sarah's copayment and her initial authorization for 4 sessions.

With a computer program and Sarah's zip code or county of residence, Rita was able to search a national database of tens of thousands of therapists for the female professionals closest to Sarah who reported specializing in anxiety disorders. There were probably at least a hundred names on the network within 15 miles of Sarah's zip code alone.

How many choices does a client get? In terms of the number of names to be given a patient who calls for a referral, it is generally common practice that patients will be furnished with three to five names from which to choose, unless the patient lives in an underserved area. However, NCQA (1998, 2000) does not specify a minimum number of names that should be offered a client requesting a referral.

The large MBHOs do not routinely make directories available to their "covered lives," nor is there any accreditation or government entity requiring them to do so.

Why not the entire list? The fact that Sarah needed to call in the first place to get the names of participating therapists is where mental health differs radically from managed medical care. The medical plans publish annual directories of their primary care physicians and network specialists, which are distributed each year at open enrollment. However, the large MBHOs do not routinely make directories available to their "covered lives," nor is there any accreditation or government entity requiring them to do so. Even purchasers of benefits don't always agree with this policy. *Managed Care Strategies* (1998) quoted a benefit plan manager who was not happy about companies' refusal to publish lists of their participating therapists. Managed behavioral care companies typically offer several reasons for their refusal to print directories, but logic alone can refute most of these claims.

Network fluidity is one such reason for no directories. But why not do what most medical plans that publish directories do? They prominently display a disclaimer stating that the consumer must verify the doctor's network participation with the insurance company to assure coverage at in-network rates.

"Clients are assured of precertification if they have to call to get names of therapists." This is what I was told to tell clients when they asked why there was no directory. But why would a managed care company want clients to precertify? Wouldn't they instead want fewer clients to precertify, so that they could save money on claims? Nor is this even true. A client like Sarah, who calls to get names, must call back to precertify once she has selected a therapist. If Sarah does not, she has not precertified.

Do the companies just not want to assume the expense of printing directories? This, too, is illogical. Whatever the expenses involved in producing directories, the vastly decreased call volume from members wanting names translates into fewer staff who have to be paid to give out names over the phone, and is almost certain to offset the directory-production costs.

Dr. Griffith of Magellan explained managed care's viewpoint: Not publishing directories is a *value-added* service. "There isn't a lot of understanding among laypeople regarding how to choose a mental health provider. We think that's a value we can add to the process for the consumer. A directory would make it more likely people will pick a name at random. It's a service-driven reason."

However, the most obvious problem with the need to call the managed behavioral care company and be assessed by an intake clinician is the immediate loss of the consumer's confidentiality (see Chapter 6). The *value-added* argument also reveals a fundamental disrespect of the consumer of psychotherapy services. People needing psychotherapy have many methods available in their communities to educate themselves about obtaining mental health/substance abuse services. They were able to find therapists successfully before the days of managed care. Friends, neighbors, clergy, primary care physicians, teachers, coworkers, and so on, are natural resources. There's also the Internet, which is a powerful tool and has many

The most obvious problem with the need to call the managed behavioral care company and be assessed by an intake clinician is the immediate loss of the consumer's confidentiality.

useful informational sites focusing on mental health issues and the kinds of treatment which are available.

Not distributing directories with the names of all participating professionals ensures that the managed care company retains maximum control over who gets the majority of referrals.

Not distributing directories with the names of all participating professionals ensures that the managed care company retains maximum control over who gets the majority of referrals. This, too, is typically considered a *value-added* service: the managed care company is "managing" the care by steering the client to a therapist who is known, through specialty credentialing and *provider-profiling,* to be the right specialist for a client presenting with a particular issue.

Who Gets the Referrals?

When faced with a list of more than about 5 names in the managed care company's database, the triage clinician or customer service rep must make choices regarding which therapist's name and phone number to give to the client. How do they make these choices?

It's not completely alphabetical anymore. In earlier days, the software returned lists of therapists per zip code in alphabetical order. Therapists whose last name began with W, were thus "alphabetically challenged" in terms of the likelihood of receiving referrals from the managed care company. Now, the databases are organized in more sophisticated ways, according to the various measures that together are referred to as *provider-profiling* (see Chapter 3).

Factors such as the client's need for a specialist, wishes regarding gender, ethnicity, discipline, age, and geographical convenience of the therapist are the first criteria used by intake clinicians and customer service representatives.

Referrals are not strictly determined by *provider-profiling.* Factors such as the client's need for a specialist, wishes regarding gender, ethnicity, discipline, age, and geographical convenience of the therapist are the first criteria used by intake clinicians and customer service representatives. But are these employees even allowed access to the entire list of names?

Companies typically utilize only a fraction of the total number of contracted professionals on their networks. Magellan, for example, was formed from the mergers of Merit Behavioral Care (MBC), Human Affairs International (HAI), and Green Spring, which, as independent companies, were respectively ranked 2, 3, and 4 among the ten largest companies in January 1997 (Oss & Clary, 1997). Their combined network size at the time the mergers were completed was estimated at 58,000 contracted professionals nationwide, serving about 62 million "covered lives" (*Open Minds,* 1998). The AAMFT publication, *Practice*

Strategies, reported in September 1999 that "about half of nearly 60,000 contracted providers in the networks for merged Magellan Behavioral Health have gone up to a year with no new referrals." Dr. Griffith explained that, "for the foreseeable future there are going to be providers in our network who don't get referrals but we have to retain them to meet access and density standards."

Case managers I interviewed in at least three of the five largest companies of early 1999 confirmed my own experience that zip code or other search methods would display information about the therapist beyond just name, address, phone number, and specialties. One case manager said that as therapist names appeared on the screen, the average case manager rating (see Chapter 3) was included. At two other companies, the type of contract (discounted fee-for-service, capitated, or case rate) was featured. Those with risk contracts were listed ahead of comparable professionals with fee-for-service contracts (see Chapter 15). One company had assigned name ratings such as "preferred," and were listed in the exact order that, if the company had its way, would be the order of referral preference. Case managers uniformly commented that it was unclear to them exactly how these rankings were determined.

Regardless of the company, the case managers reported having been given stern instructions never to tell contracted professionals what their rating was, or even to acknowledge that there was such a system. Their general consensus about the system was decidedly negative. One case manager said bluntly, "I have a problem with this. It seems so arbitrary." All confided that regardless of management's instructions regarding using therapists of higher rankings or certain types of contracts, their choices of names to give as referrals were primarily motivated by client preference, geographical location, and/or other clinical issues as revealed by their telephone assessment. The methods used by each company to enforce clinician compliance with the rules ranged from nonexistent to highly structured (i.e., written explanations of why certain professionals/facilities were chosen over others).

Solo Practitioners versus Groups

It's a scary economic climate; there's a lot more supply than demand in most markets, driving down the fees (see Chapter 14). Then there's capitation, which favors groups. Once an insurer or managed care company has signed a capitated contract with a group, the group runs the show,

Case managers uniformly commented that it was unclear to them exactly how these rankings were determined.

All confided that regardless of management's instructions regarding using therapists of higher rankings or certain types of contracts, their choices of names to give as referrals were primarily motivated by client preference, geographical location, and/or other clinical issues as revealed by their telephone assessment.

since they pay for all covered, "medically necessary" services (see Chapter 15). Often, clients accessing their mental health and/or substance abuse benefits never call the managed care company at all. The number printed on their insurance card leads directly to the group practice. This is one basis for the fears that solo practitioners will be completely eclipsed for any and all clients wishing to use their insurance to pay for therapy.

The experts who periodically sound the death knell for solo practice have said that eventually managed care would refuse to contract with solos, but so far they have been wrong. Although there are many reasons why managed care does prefer groups, their networks still list thousands of individual therapists. Why? The managed care companies simply haven't been able to do it; even after a decade of managed care there are not enough group practices in most markets to meet 100 percent of the demand for services.

Why not? There are many reasons why groups haven't yet achieved the level of market penetration that would be needed to shut out the solos completely. Most of these have to do with macro-level economic factors. The most obvious reason is that the expenses needed to establish and maintain group practice infrastructures that can support capitation are very high. Groups that hope to be able to contract directly with employers, or which subcontract from insurance/managed care companies on a capitated basis, must have the ability to manage services as well as deliver them. This gets into things like quality improvement and NCQA compliance (if not outright accreditation), developing utilization review and appeals systems, intake, triage and after-hours systems, outcome and satisfaction measurements, and so on. In the largest groups, these forces sometimes affect the work lives of direct-practice clinicians in ways which are perceived negatively, and people leave to begin solo practices. If there aren't enough groups, managed care has little choice but to retain solos on the network. Ultimately, whether solos are "shut out" depends on the characteristics of the local market.

Groups that hope to be able to contract directly with employers, or which subcontract from insurance/ managed care companies on a capitated basis, must have the ability to manage services as well as deliver them.

Ultimately, whether solos are "shut out" depends on the characteristics of the local market.

Appointment Accessibility

After referral, managed care companies expect that the patient will be seen within a certain period of time, depending on the clinical urgency of the situation as assessed by the managed care company's intake clinician. *Appointment accessibility* is one of the most common specific *provider-profiling* measures. It's also a frequently-used quality indicator and focus of performance guarantees. When clients are discharged from inpatient or other higher levels of mental health/substance abuse care, the number of days until their first follow-up outpatient appointment is also closely watched; it's a HEDIS® measure (see Chapter 1).

Timeframes for Initial Appointments

NCQA (2000, QI 5) specifies assessment of clients into one of four categories: *emergent-life threatening, emergent-not life threatening, urgent,* or *routine. Emergent* situations require immediate attention and generally result in clients being referred to a hospital or facility for evaluation. *Urgent* clients, on the other hand, are often expected to be initially assessed as outpatients. (See Table 5.1.)

Clinicians and/or nonclinical support staff will make as many calls as they have to in order to find an appointment for a client assessed as *emergent* or *urgent.*

Assessing Urgency. If the phone is initially answered by a nonclinician, they will probably ask the client a few high-risk screening questions. If the client answers yes, or if there is any doubt, the call is then sent to a licensed clinician. There is usually a checklist, published internally for reference and documentation purposes, which guides the clinician performing telephone triage and who is making the determination (Table 5.2). The specific issues and/or situations which constitute *emergent* versus *urgent* are defined by each managed behavioral care company, *not* by the NCQA.

Most typically, *emergent* means a life-threatening situation, or one that may become life-threatening without immediate intervention. *Urgent*

> *Clinicians and/or nonclinical support staff will make as many calls as they have to in order to find an appointment for a client assessed as emergent or urgent.*
>
> *The specific issues and/or situations which constitute emergent versus urgent are defined by each managed behavioral care company, not by the NCQA.*

Table 5.1
NCQA Timeframes for Initial Appointments

Assessment	Maximum Wait Time
Emergent, life threatening	Immediately
Emergent, non-life threatening	6 hours
Urgent	48 hours
Routine	10 business days

Outpatient follow-up after discharge from a higher level of care: within 30 days

Source: NCQA, 2000, Q 5.1.1–5.1.4; NCQA, 1998 HEDIS 3.0.

Table 5.2
Emergent or Just Plain Urgent?*

Issue	Emergent	Urgent
Suicidality	Client indicates ready availability of lethal means Client indicates present intent to harm self No social support system available to help client remain safe Client using alcohol/drugs likely to impair judgment or increase risk of acting impulsively Presence of psychosis/thought disorder	Client reports thoughts of death and/or suicide, but denies ready availability of lethal means Client denies present intent to act in self-harmful manner Client has social support system available to monitor safety and withhold access to lethal means until the time of appointment Not using alcohol/drugs likely to impair judgment or increase impulsivity Absence of psychosis/thought disorder
Chemical Dependency	Pattern and amount of use likely to lead to overdose with medical complications Withdrawal syndromes (or potential withdrawal) resulting in medical complications or which could be lethal Concurrent suicidal and/or homicidal ideation/plan History of psychosis and/or dual diagnosis: drinking/using while on psychotropic medications which may require stabilization	Use not enough to risk withdrawal within the next 48 hours, or use of substances with no withdrawal lethality or few potential medical complications Available social support to refrain from drinking/using while waiting for appointment No concurrent suicidality/homicidality No concurrent psychosis or dual diagnosis requiring immediate stabilization of meds

*Each managed care company publishes its own (*proprietary*) criteria for determining *emergent, urgent,* and *routine* situations. Check with the relevant MBHO to determine their criteria. These are samples only.

means that there are serious risk factors necessitating evaluation and/or treatment as soon as possible, but that the situation is not presently life-threatening, and not likely to escalate into anything life-threatening in the next 2 days. In practice, determinations of *urgent* versus *emergent* are the judgment call of the clinician performing the telephone evaluation, in consultation with a supervisor.

Managed care employees frequently hear the protest, "But it was an emergency!" in response to their explanations that payment for the session on such-and-such date, usually an initial outpatient session, was denied due to lack of precertification. Unfortunately, managed care company staff is expected to adhere to the company's guidelines of what constitutes an *emergent* situation, not the therapist's. As a participating member of the network, the managed care company should furnish, upon written or verbal request, a copy of their criteria that distinguishes *emergent* from *urgent* or *routine* sessions. Sometimes the definition of *emergent* can actually be found in a participating-provider contract or in the Provider Manual.

If these definitions are not already available in written form in official materials, if the managed care company refuses to release them, and/or if they say there are no such definitions, consider calling the state's Department of Insurance. Depending on the client's type of benefit plan, the Department of Insurance may have the authority to arbitrate in retrospect as to whether a particular situation was or was not an emergency and should be reimbursed. Many states have now adopted *prudent layperson* standards, which, depending on the specific law, may apply to coverage of mental health emergencies.

Does the managed care company really check to see when clients had their appointments, in "routine" situations? They most certainly do. Accounts in which there are high financial targets at risk for meeting a contractual routine appointments accessibility guarantee, may employ clerks who contact clients and/or therapists to find out when they had, or will be having, their first appointments. Other times, the intake clinician who handled the client's call follows up with the client to make sure an appointment was offered within the benchmark time frame.

If clients are given names of several therapists at the time of their initial call, but didn't precertify treatment, there are various human and electronic tracking systems available which can "flag" the case for follow-up if after a certain number of days the client hasn't called back to precertify. Then the clerk(s) (or intake clinicians) get the names and make the phone calls, asking if a therapist has been chosen. Intrusive? To therapists, yes. To a managed behavioral care company, though, it's considered part of the *value-added* service: the managed care employee can both (1) facilitate precertification and (2) provide education as to the importance of treatment.

Whether or not proactive monitoring/intervening is also done by managed care staff, most managed care companies measure appointment accessibility retroactively by including it as a question on member satisfaction surveys. Some companies now also ask that professionals furnish the date/time of the first appointment offered, when they complete the first treatment report.

Depending on the client's type of benefit plan, the Department of Insurance may have the authority to arbitrate in retrospect as to whether a particular situation was or was not an emergency and should be reimbursed.

6

Adding Value,
Subtracting Privacy

Psychiatrist Fred Sigmund, MD, was tired of being pestered by drug company salespeople, but he put up with it because of the free samples. Many of his elderly patients had difficulty paying for their prescriptions, even with their insurance coverage. But something really had to be done. Just last week, one of those pushy salespeople had gone too far. The rep from WondRDrug Pharmaceuticals had consulted a computer printout, saying,

"I see here that you've prescribed Drug X for Mrs. Cartwright. May I ask why you felt this was a better choice than WondRDrug's Drug Y?"

Dr. Sigmund was speechless for a moment. How dare some drug salesperson with no medical education presume to question his prescribing? Didn't this fool know that for him to discuss the matter was a violation of the patient's confidentiality?

Dr. Sigmund decided that free samples or no, he was not going to put up with this. He coldly explained to the WondRDrug rep that to discuss the matter would be a violation of confidentiality and that he had no intention of helping a company that would stoop to such levels to make a profit.

A month later, Mrs. Cartwright asked Dr. Sigmund why he had prescribed Drug X for her rather than Drug Y. Remembering the incident with the drug rep, Dr. Sigmund asked Mrs. Cartwright the reason for her question. Mrs. Cartwright said, "I received this brochure in the mail," and pulled out of her purse some literature which had been sent to her by WondRDrug Pharmaceuticals.

Any time the payer of psychotherapy is other than the patient, that payer will require information to justify continuing to pay, and there is loss of confidentiality.

The confidential medical and psychological information of anyone who has ever used insurance benefits for any reason is "out there." Any time the payer of psychotherapy is other than the patient, that payer will require information to justify continuing to pay, and there is loss of confidentiality.

Who Can Access the Confidential Information?

Norman Hering, MFT, is a former case manager at a national MBHO. He has appeared on the *20/20* television news program and is active in the California Coalition for Ethical Mental Health Care (CCEMHC) and the American Mental Health Alliance (AMHA). In our interview, Hering stated, "Practically everyone in the company had access to the care management computer system, which contained the clinical information."

Practically everyone in the company had access to the care management computer system, which contained the clinical information.

Customer Service and Claims Reps

Whether customer service and claims reps can actually read clinical information such as diagnosis, problems, treatment plan, or what practitioners said on outpatient treatment reports depends on the design specifications of the company's information system. Does access to the benefits, eligibility, claims, and authorization portions of the computerized record carry with it the ability to read about the client's problem, diagnosis, and treatment plan? In my experience, the answer was frequently *yes.*

What about the risks of nonclinical personnel having access to confidential information who may not understand the finer points of maintaining confidentiality? Take spouses, for instance. Anyone who can give the customer service rep a patient birthdate, address, and/or a social security number might receive information to which he or she might not be entitled. As Hering (1999) states, "A clinician knows that a spouse does not have a right to access records and would require a release of information. A nonclinical staff member might disclose inappropriate information in a naïve attempt to be helpful."

Anyone who can give the customer service rep a patient birthdate, address, and/or a social security number might receive information to which he or she might not be entitled.

Data Entry/Other Nonclinical Support Staff in the Care Management Department

Clinical material is frighteningly integral to the jobs of these employees. They collect the faxes from the machines, open the mail, route treatment reports to the appropriate case manager, and, at some companies, microfilm the treatment plans before they are reviewed. They may be responsible for typing the clinical information word-for-word into the computer system prior to the review by the case manager. Bachelors' level staff at some companies may actually review outpatient treatment reports, in some cases (see Chapter 8).

Although the managed care companies claim they train their nonclinician employees, and despite the fact that they are made to sign confidentiality agreements upon hire, how can anyone really be sure?

Provider Relations/Network

There are two reasons managed care companies justify allowing the Provider Relations and the Network Department access to the clinical information system. The first is for *provider-profiling* (see Chapter 3). The other reason given is that investigations of client complaints about practitioners often need to be taken in the clinical context of the patient who made the complaint. Network management employees use the electronic case record as one source of information to investigate patient complaints. Some of these employees have clinical backgrounds, others do not.

Account Management

Account executives are often involved in denials, unusual or high-profile requests for treatment (such as experimental or long-term residential care), and complaints, particularly from the employer's VIPs. All of which may require information about a particular case to aid in the resolution process. Additionally, account executives work with the Quality Improvement Department on preparing reports and audits, and the data for these reports originates, at least in part, from the clinical information system.

Quality Improvement

Quality Improvement (QI) (or QA, for Quality Assurance) randomly audits patient files to assure compliance with NCQA, other accreditation organizations, internal company standards, and contractual performance guarantees made to employers (see Chapter 1). If, for example, a promise has been made that 95 percent of outpatients with primary or secondary diagnoses of substance abuse will be referred to 12-step groups, the QI reviewers will have the computer generate a random sample of patients, then search each record for the appropriate documentation.

Information Systems

IS staff obviously have to be able to access every computer platform, network, and any software packages used by company employees, in order to maintain functionality and perform necessary upgrades. They are also responsible for implementing and maintaining intact whatever "firewalls" (barriers) exist between the company's computer system and the outside world.

Another concern about the computer systems in use by the large managed care companies is noted by Pomerantz (1999c): most if not all of the companies file clinical and authorization information by social security number. Anyone with a social security number can potentially gain access, and social security numbers are easy to obtain. How does the managed care company know whether the caller is truly who he or she says, if they have the right social security number? A few customer service reps will take the extra step of asking for confirmation of a birthdate or address (also relatively easy information to obtain), but none use a PIN number, special encrypted account number, or code word to prevent disclosures to anyone but the client.

Access to Other Accounts

The universality of access is also an issue, regardless of an employee's job classification. Do employees have access to records from accounts other than the ones with which they work? Often, yes, and this is also an issue of information-system design.

Prospective Customers

Bea Worker, case manager at GenRUs Behavioral Health (GBH), worked in one of the larger service centers. The general-distribution voice mail she received one Friday afternoon, therefore, did not come as any great surprise. It was from one of the secretaries to the director of the service center, announcing the visit the following week of a very important prospective customer.

"This is just a reminder that we are proud to host executives from Southern Regional Bank Conglomerate on Monday and Tuesday of next week. Please have your work areas clean and presentable, and remember to wear business attire. Thank you for your cooperation, and have a nice weekend."

It's a familiar drill to anyone working in a major regional or national managed care office. Groups of executives from companies considering contracting visit, are given tours, and one of the main attractions always is the case management unit(s). Nor is this even a rare event; visits from one employer or another occurred at least once or twice monthly.

Norman Hering commented that the prospective customers were allowed free access to the areas in which the case managers worked, and in some cases even sat with case managers, watching them do their jobs. In my experience, the intake units were the most vulnerable to such displays, and the VIPs would watch supervisors take calls. The potential confidentiality loss is obvious—and disturbing. Hering agreed, saying, "It's virtually impossible to protect confidentiality." How can anyone be sure that the VIPs won't hear names of clients, or glimpse names on computer screens or paper documents as they pass by?

One wonders why the visiting employers don't realize that, if they sign this contract, their employees and families are likely to be the next ones to lose confidentiality.

No Confidentiality of Participation

Confidentiality isn't just about content of therapy, presenting problems, treatment plan, or diagnosis—but the very participation in therapy itself. Even classes of MBHO employees not allowed direct access to the clinical information system, are still likely to come across client names at any time.

If there were reliable indicators of how well companies adhere to their policies in practice, clinicians would be able to use these as guides to pick and choose the ethical companies with which to work.

Policy versus Practice: How Is Confidentiality Handled inside the Managed Care Company?

The corporate policy outlined in an official three-ring binder in the CEO's office might not have much resemblance to the daily operations of the managed care company. All the managed care companies claim that the issue of confidentiality is treated with the highest respect and is given top priority, to ensure the most stringent safeguards of sensitive information possible. If this is true, then they should have no reason to object to the scrutiny of their policies and actual practices by the professional community as well as the accreditation organizations. If there were reliable indicators of how well companies adhere to their policies in practice, clinicians would be able to use these as guides to pick and choose the ethical companies with which to work.

They Site Visit Us . . . Why Not the Other Way Around?

When was the last time any of the national professional organizations or state chapters site-visited a local managed care company office and checked out the confidentiality aspects of the operation with a critical eye? We professionals can do a lot more than we currently do to force the issue of confidentiality into the forefront.

Managed care companies and NCQA publish criteria for use when site-visiting therapists' offices (see Chapter 4). In this spirit, Figure 6.1 offers guidelines for evaluating managed care company operations if professional association representatives or individual practitioners do go inside for a visit.

The area of confidentiality safeguards can be quite technical when it comes to things like computers, the Internet, electronic mail, voice mail, and telephone monitoring systems. Professional associations might consider hiring a technical/computer consultant to evaluate the mechanisms put in place by the companies to ensure security.

Getting Away with Breaking Confidentiality

What if a nonclinical employee of a managed care company breaches confidentiality? An administrative assistant or customer service rep doesn't have a professional license to lose. What consequences would this person face for their actions? Would the company even take responsibility?

Common sense would seem to indicate that the company should be legally liable for the maintenance of confidentiality by its employees. Certainly therapists in private practice who hire secretaries, office managers and so forth have always paid higher premiums on their malpractice insurance to cover the risk of breach of confidentiality by an employee. Bernstein and Hartsell (1998), both lawyers, state unequivocally that therapists are responsible for breaches of confidentiality by their employees. Shouldn't this also be true for managed care companies or large corporate healthcare entities?

Figure 6.1
Checklist for Evaluation of Managed Care Company Confidentiality Practices

1. *Do the case managers lock their papers up each night or shred them to avoid prying eyes?* Examine the physical layout. Do the cubes have file drawers that lock? What is on the desks? Can anyone start up the case manager's computer, or is it password-protected? Is there a password-protected screen saver for when the case manager is away from his or her desk?

2. *What employees are allowed into the area where the clinical work is done?* Consider the following categories of employees: appeals, claims, customer service, QI, sales, account management, finance/purchasing, network/provider relations, info systems/technical, maintenance or janitorial, human resources, executive, administrative, data entry/transcriptionists, corporate security personnel.

3. *Are there security measures in place to bar physical access by unauthorized personnel?* (i.e., locked doors requiring electronic ID card or other similar measure)

4. *Are materials with confidential client information allowed to leave the area where the clinical work is done?* (If yes, is there any procedure for tracking who has what? How does this procedure work?)

5. *How does the company ensure that nonclinical employees maintain standards of confidentiality when or if, in the course of their jobs, they come across names, identifying information, diagnoses, and /or case summaries?* What training is held for nonclinical employees and supervisors on the issue of confidentiality? How often? Is the trainer a clinician? Do nonclinical employees have ready access to a clinician if they have a question about whether or not to reveal information? What, if any, job penalties or disciplinary actions are there for breaches of confidentiality by nonclinical personnel?

6. *What sorts of QI initiatives are there to tighten confidentiality?* Are there frequent and random internal confidentiality audits? Is there someone on each relevant work team designated to act as "confidentiality police?"

7. *Who can access electronic mail, U.S. postal mail, paper files, faxes, and voice mail, as well as computerized clinical records?* Who collects the faxes from the machines? Can supervisors or other employees access voice mailboxes, or stored electronic mail? Are there cross-cut paper shredders at various locations in the office (i.e., near copiers, fax machines, and near the clinical workstations)? Ask technical details about how the safeguards work and how the company arranges it so that access is as limited as possible.

8. *Computer security.* If a case manager or nonclinical employee with access to clinical information is working exclusively on Company X's benefit plan, can this employee access any information about the employees or family members from Companies Y or Z whose mental health benefits are also managed by the organization? What, if any, safeguards are there which shield the clinical information from customer service reps, claims processors, and all other nonclinician employees whose jobs do not require access to it?

9. *Does the company maintain hard copy or microfilm records?* How and where are they stored? Who has access? Are records ever allowed to leave the storage area? Who is allowed to check them out? Are there strict procedures regarding return of borrowed materials?

10. *Telephone monitoring.* Who has access to live telephone monitoring systems? Are calls recorded? If so, are these recordings kept? Who listens to them?

Just ask "Jane Doe," of Albany, New York, about her experiences with Kaiser-Community Health Plan (CHP). In 1997, Jane sought psychotherapy with a social worker employed by CHP. Jane later heard from a coworker that a file clerk at Kaiser-CHP, Christen Adey, had reportedly told a group of Jane's coworkers that she was a lesbian, a fact Adey read in the chart. Jane subsequently sued Kaiser-CHP. From a therapist's point of view, the outcome of the suit should have been a no-brainer. However, the court ruled in favor of Kaiser-CHP, saying that because Adey was not acting in furtherance of her duties when she released the information, the company could not be held liable (Grace, 1999).

How can this be? According to Jane Doe's attorney, Lee Greenstein, "there is no direct statute in New York concerning employer liability for breach of confidentiality by [non-professional] employees" (personal communication, May 7, 1999). Greenstein further indicated that in depositions, Ms. Adey admitted to breaking Jane's confidentiality, and said that there had been no training by Kaiser-CHP on the issue of confidentiality, just a request to sign a confidentiality agreement.

Judge Joseph Teresi, in the written ruling, decried the decision he was obligated to make because of the inadequacy of the law:

> with the availability of extremely intimate and historically protected information now at the hands of many as the file works its way through the maze of the health care infrastructure, it appears that, in reality, this information is in fact unchaperoned by adequate confidentiality. It appears reasonable that an employer, who knows his employees will have access to this type of information, be held to more exacting standards than the present law allows. (*Jane Doe vs. Kaiser-CHP & Adey*, 1999)

Incidentally, despite her admission of having broken confidentiality, Kaiser-CHP did not fire Adey until the day after the judge's decision—two years after the original incident. Says Greenstein, "I think it's an indication of how little regard they have for confidentiality."

What's the Lesson to Be Learned?

As professionals who are routinely obligated to release sensitive clinical information for the purposes of payment, it behooves us to find out what the laws are that regulate the conduct of managed care companies in maintaining confidentiality. The implication of *Jane Doe vs. Kaiser-CHP & Adey* seems to be that if companies go through the merest show of

The implication of Jane Doe vs. Kaiser-CHP & Adey seems to be that if companies go through the merest show of "training" and documenting confidentiality policies and procedures, they can evade liability when the inevitable happens.

"training" and documenting confidentiality policies and procedures, they can evade liability when the inevitable happens. Through professional associations and grassroots organizations, we therapists can be active in helping to strengthen the laws and press for the right to inspect the actual practices of managed care companies.

Lee Greenstein summarized the situation neatly, commenting, "If they aren't held accountable there's no incentive for HMOs to hold things confidential. Keeping records confidential was a job function of this clerk and she violated it."

Managed Care "Products"

When I was employed as a case manager, one of the company's most important contracts came up for renewal and the corporate customer decided to solicit bids from other companies. This was a large and influential employer, with the contract valued at millions of dollars. A shaken-looking senior executive called an emergency meeting of the entire team. The essence of the executive's presentation was focused on how we had to demonstrate quality to the employer, in preparation for our company's rebidding on the contract. The actual words used rang in my head as an alarming admission for someone in this executive's position to make: "Managed care services take away from dollars available for treatment. We're like a parasite on the mental health delivery system. Therefore, we have to demonstrate the value of our services to [the employer]."

The phrase *value-added* is the theme song of managed care: Companies justify their very existence with it. Their salespeople market products such as a full telephone clinical intake, case management, using the continuum of care effectively to achieve the twin goals of maximized treatment effectiveness and cost savings, disability management, and so on. While there is no question that these services are an enhancement, the *value-added* infrastructure is expensive and has one other fundamental weakness: an inherent loss of privacy. The *value-added* intake process serves as a case in point.

While there is no question that these services are an enhancement, the value-added infrastructure is expensive and has one other fundamental weakness: an inherent loss of privacy.

The Value-Added Intake Process

When a managed care company requires the patient to be responsible for precertification, it's usually because the intake process was sold as being *value-added*, meaning that the customer was promised that members would be guided to the most appropriate practitioner and level of care for the presenting issue. To determine what is most "appropriate," naturally, requires clinical assessment by the managed care company's intake staff. Thus, clients are thrust into a position of having lost their confidentiality before they ever step foot inside a therapist's office. Depending on the specific company and the provisions of the benefit plan, authorization of sessions may be denied or reimbursement reduced if clients refuse to participate in this process.

What do intake clinicians ask? Anything a therapist would ask in an initial therapy session. An *audit checklist* is typically used by supervisory and/or QI staff to make certain that the assessments (and subsequent documentation) are as thorough as possible (Figure 6.2).

Is all this really necessary? What if the client just wants to use the EAP?

Nelson Lawrence, LPC, intake clinician for HPBH, received a call from a client who indicated she wanted to see an EAP therapist. The client, Maryanne Meade, when asked what the situation was, explained that she was being stalked by a much older man with whom she'd briefly been involved. She was now in a new relationship with a man her own age, and wanted to be free of "this pervert." Maryanne sounded anxious and agitated. She denied problems in other life areas, substance abuse, and suicidal/homicidal ideation or plan. Nelson referred her to the closest female EAP counselor.

Nelson's notes in the system contained only the following information: "24-year-old female, briefly involved with older man, now in new relationship but older man is stalking. Anxious WNL. Denies SA, SI/HI, depressive symptoms, or work impairments. Indicates willingness to take appropriate action (i.e., calling police) as needed. Referred to Dina Troy, LCSW as requested for EAP & benefit of 6 sessions entered in system. Called & left message with Ms. Troy's answering service re: new referral."

Nelson's supervisor, Evonne Brown, listened to this conversation and read his documentation as part of HPBH's continuous quality improvement process. She gave him an "Unacceptable" score of 80 percent, citing:

- Failure to ask "appropriate and necessary" history questions about Maryanne's past mental health/substance abuse treatment;

- Failure to ask "appropriate and necessary" questions about any medical problems Maryanne might have and/or medications prescribed;

- Failure to ask for details about the stalking. (i.e., was he calling her? following her in his car?);

Figure 6.2
Intake Assessment Audit Checklist

Date: _____   Clinician: _____

Telephone call audit or Record review   Clinician Score: _____

Scoring: 0 = N/A, 1 = absent, 2 = some attempt to ask/document but effort is incomplete, 3 = satisfactory,
4 = outstanding

For Telephone Audit Only:

_____ Positive, professional demeanor   _____ Listened effectively
_____ Explained benefits   _____ Answered questions fully
_____ Explained confidentiality   _____ Did not interrupt
_____ Asked about patient's choice regarding provider gender,   _____ Gave at least 3 referral choices
        discipline, racial/cultural background   _____ Puts patient at ease
_____ If patient wanted out-of-network provider, offered in-network
        choices
_____ If patient did not accept referral, reminded patient to call back   Subtotal: _____
        to precertify
_____ Asked at the end of the call if patient got what he or she needed/is
        there anything else you need?

For Telephone Audit and/or Record Review:
_____ Clinician asks/Documents reason for seeking treatment at this particular time.
_____ Clinician asks/Documents specific precipitant to today's call for help.
_____ Clinician asks/Documents patient's goals for treatment.
_____ Clinician asks/Documents assessment of patient's strengths.
_____ Clinician asks/Documents assessment of patient's obstacles to achieving goals.
_____ Clinician asks/Documents presenting symptoms.
_____ Clinician asks/Documents impairments in functioning.
_____ Clinician asks/Documents immediate threats to safety of patient and others (suicide, homicide, domestic
        violence, child/elder abuse).
        _____ If immediate risk factors are present, clinician asks/Documents imminent plan and/or intent.
        _____ If immediate risk factors are present, clinician asks/Documents presence of firearms/other means.
        _____ If immediate risk factors are present, clinician asks/Documents past history of this and all other
                risk factors.
        _____ If immediate risk factors are present, clinician asks/Documents available social support.
        _____ If immediate risk factors are present, clinician develops and documents safety plan with caller and
                collateral social support.
        _____ If immediate risk factors are present and no plan can be developed, clinician consults with super-
                visor and calls police if directed to do so.
                                                                      Subtotal: _____

Figure 6.2 (Continued)

_____ Clinician asks/Documents substance abuse:

_____ Substance(s) used	_____ Age of first use	_____ Amounts used in last
_____ Prescription drug assessment	_____ Length of use	24–48 hours
	_____ 12-step participation	_____ Previous overdoses
_____ Family history	_____ Job consequences	_____ History of withdrawal,
_____ Previous treatment	_____ Amounts used on a	DT's, seizures
_____ Legal consequences	regular basis	
_____ Method of use		

Subtotal: _____

_____ Clinician asks/Documents previous mental health treatment:

_____ Date of previous treatment	_____ Provider/Facility
_____ Level of care	_____ Problem(s) for which treatment was sought
_____ Outcome	

Subtotal: _____

_____ Clinician asks/Documents nature of family and social support system.
_____ Clinician asks/Documents nature of job functioning/problems.
_____ If patient is child/adolescent, clinician asks/Documents nature of school functioning/problems.
_____ If patient is child/adolescent, clinician asks/Documents nature of peer relationships/problems.
_____ If patient is child/adolescent, clinician asks/Documents nature of family relationships/problems.
_____ If patient is child/adolescent, clinician asks/Documents presence of prenatal/perinatal complications.
_____ Clinician asks/Documents medical issues.
_____ Clinician asks/Documents medications prescribed.

Subtotal: _____

Certification:

_____ All five axes of diagnosis completed.	_____ Explanation of why level of care meets medical necessity criteria, citing specific criteria.
_____ Diagnosis follows from presenting problems/symptoms.	_____ Patient referred to provider with documented specialty (if appropriate).
_____ Clinician documented call to provider notifying of referral and certification.	_____ Treatment goals documented.

Subtotal: _____

- Failure to tell Maryanne to go directly to the police; and
- Failure to ask about problems at work.

From a managed care, *value-added* perspective, there is a need for all these questions. In this case, the client may be in danger from the stalker; other times, clients might be suicidal or self-injurious. Maryanne might have a need for more than the 6 EAP sessions allowed by her company. Thorough assessment enables the clinician to make a better determination as to the appropriate level of care and intervene with the client to protect safety in addition to making the referral. Thus, the "product" sold by the managed are organization is in fundamental conflict with most clinicians' value of privacy.

Audit checklists serve as a guide to the intake clinician in knowing what to ask. The checklist is then scored, and serves as a measure for evaluating the intake clinician's competence at his or her job. Is it fair to expect clinicians whose jobs depend on satisfactory audit scores to refuse to ask intrusive questions on ethical grounds? Who should set the standard regarding what constitutes "too intrusive" on the part of a managed care entity?

Is it worth it? What the client reveals during the *value-added* intake then goes into the same computerized record as the information from therapists' treatment reports. Then there's the issue of client's rights in situations where the *value-added* assessment is mandatory in order to obtain benefit coverage. Shouldn't there be a basic right of clients to have a benefit-covered, in-person assessment with the therapist of their choice, by-passing the managed care company's intake process?

Predetermining the Cost of Treatment

"Diversion" is a re-directing of the patient to a level of care lower, cheaper, or shorter than that which was originally requested, based on an evaluation by someone employed by or directly contracted with the insurer/managed care company.

Value-added intake serves as a clear example of managed care companies' ability to justify what also serves their financial interests. The intake clinician is usually asked to document in the electronic record how many sessions he or she thinks the client will need to complete treatment. This assessment is expected to aid the utilization review case manager.

Corporate expectations in the form of the ubiquitous performance guarantees (see Chapter 1) and the ability to increase profits, likewise, may color the intake clinician's determination as to "appropriate" level of care. For example, the client may be assessed by the intake clinician as needing medication, and sent to a psychiatrist, even if talk therapy was requested. Such a maneuver is a "diversion," that is, re-directing the patient to a level of care lower, cheaper, or shorter than that which was originally requested, based on an evaluation by someone employed by or directly contracted with the insurer/managed care company.

Diversions

Diverting is a classic managed care tactic which occurs at the point of intake. In the early days of managed care, it was primarily used to control the number of inpatient admissions. For example, a patient requesting mental health or substance abuse treatment shows up unexpectedly at the emergency room or treatment center. Instead of being evaluated by hospital staff who then call the managed care company for precertification, the company sends out an employee, contracted practitioner, or a clinician from a local contracted crisis-response team, to do the assessment. The goal of the diversion assessment is to find that the medical necessity for treatment at the requested level of care is not sufficient.

The goal of the diversion assessment is to find that the medical necessity for treatment at the requested level of care is not sufficient.

Diversions may also occur as a result of the *value-added* intake process. For example, a client calls, requesting outpatient therapy, but instead is sent to an EAP. Some EAPs do not allow *self-referral*, that is, it is contractually forbidden to continue to see the client and use outpatient managed mental health benefits when the EAP sessions are used up. The client must then choose between starting all over with a benefit-covered outpatient therapist, or paying out-of-pocket to continue to see the EAP therapist. Clients who develop a relationship with their EAP therapist and choose to continue their therapy by paying out-of-pocket, are a savings to the managed care company, particularly one which operates under an *at-risk* contract (see Chapter 7).

To the client, where is the value for which privacy has been sacrificed? Does the value of the service provided by the managed care company outweigh the traditional value of privacy in mental health and substance abuse treatment? Are there other methods of managing utilization at the point of intake that do not impair privacy? These are important considerations as managed care undergoes a period of evolution and increased regulation.

Empowerment

As therapists participating in the managed care system, we can help clients empower themselves to take back control of the intake/precertification process and preserve as much of their privacy as possible. The way to help clients empower themselves is to teach them how the system operates.

The way to help clients empower themselves is to teach them how the system operates.

Educate your clients! You don't have to answer all those questions. *For EAP,* you have the right to see a therapist, regardless of the issues you wish to discuss, because your employer has prepaid for you to use this service. By definition, EAP services do not have to be "medically necessary." *For managed care,* find out if your benefit plan allows pass-through sessions, or if your state mandates a certain number of these sessions. If you aren't entitled to pass-through sessions, answer the questions as briefly as possible. Feel free to ask the intake clinician, "What happens to this information?" and "Why are you asking this?" Or, consider paying for the first few sessions privately, to discuss the issues with your therapist, before precertifying.

Brochures written for the consumer are available from most professional and advocacy associations (see Resources appendix). Clients participating in the *value-added* intake process need to know and understand that they have rights, and be able to assert themselves. Therapists who suspect that their clients are not able to assert themselves adequately when dealing with "the system" may want to consider having the client call from the office, where they can be on hand to offer support and direction.

Alternatives to Value-Added Intake

With the pass-through session method, the managed care company will automatically authorize a given number sessions to the client, regardless of the presenting diagnosis or problems.

Some companies use *pass-through sessions* to return the comprehensive assessment function to the therapist. With the pass-through session method, the managed care company will automatically authorize a given number sessions to the client, regardless of the presenting diagnosis or problems. There is no mandate for members to engage in detailed telephone assessments with intake clinicians employed by the managed care company. (*"Pass through" sessions are not the same as an EAP. Unlike an EAP, "pass-throughs" are not free to the client; whatever copayment is required by the benefit plan must be paid.*) Precertification, sometimes called case registration, simply is a matter of informing the managed care company that therapy will be beginning between a covered member and an in-network therapist, and can be done either by the client, the therapist, or the therapist's office staff.

Depending on the number of "pass-throughs" allowed by the benefit plan, some clients with less severe problems may even be able to end treatment within their pass-through sessions, which means that the only information in their file is a diagnosis, supplied by the therapist on the claims. Clients whose therapy is not completed, may decide to self-pay after the "pass-throughs" end. "Pass-throughs" also furnish clients with the opportunity to discuss with their therapist the pros and cons of going through "medical necessity" determinations that will obtain further benefit coverage but result in loss of privacy. One factor in this decision may be the total benefit financial benefit left to the client after the "pass-throughs" have been used.

The benefit = The discounted fee, minus the copayment, multiplied by the number of sessions

For number of sessions, take the maximum amount allowed per year, but explain to the client that managed care companies don't always authorize clients to use all their benefits.

So, for example, the total mental health benefit of a patient seeing a masters'-level therapist with a contracted fee of $50, a copayment of $20, and 20 sessions per year is:

$$\$50 - \$20 = \$30 \text{ per session}$$
$$\$30 \text{ multiplied by 20 sessions} = \$600$$

The "pass-through" idea is catching on. Managed Health Network (part of Foundation Health Systems) uses "pass-through" sessions for several of its accounts. Other companies, such as ValueOptions, have developed similar systems working in conjunction with professional organizations, in this case the New York State Psychological Association. According to Gayle O'Brien, director of Legal and Regulatory Affairs of the New York State Psychological Association (NYSPA), representatives from the two organizations have met quarterly since 1995. In the fall of 1998, when ValueOptions was awarded the behavioral health contract for New York State employees and their families, NYSPA was influential in getting ValueOptions to raise the number of "pass-through" sessions from 5 to 10.

Some states, such as New Hampshire, have adopted laws in this area either independently or as part of their mental health parity measures. New Hampshire's utilization review law (House bill 446, became law on 6/19/95), requires five "pass-through" sessions: two for diagnosis and three for treatment, before any utilization review is allowed to occur.

Therapists as individuals (and through our professional organizations, where it does not violate anti-trust law) can take the lead in critically examining managed care products.

Therapists as individuals (and through our professional organizations, where it does not violate anti-trust law) can take the lead in critically examining managed care products. We can make choices whose networks to serve on, and which to resign from, based on knowledgeable review of companies' policies and procedures.

Capitated systems are another way that the *value-added* services presently conducted by managed care can be returned to the professionals, and privacy restored, although capitation comes with its own set of uncomfortable issues (see Chapter 15).

7

Medical Necessity

"I've never yet heard a good definition of medical necessity."
—Case manager at one of the Big Five MBHOs

A managed care company president was given a ticket for a performance of Schubert's Unfinished Symphony. Since she was unable to go, she passed the invitation to one of her reviewers. The next morning, the president asked him how he enjoyed it, and, instead of a few plausible observations, she was handed a memorandum that read as follows:

1. For a considerable period, the oboe players had nothing to do. Their number should be reduced, and their work spread over the whole orchestra, thus avoiding peaks of inactivity.
2. All twelve violins were playing identical notes. This seems unnecessary duplication, and the staff of this section should be drastically cut. If a large volume of sound is really required, this could be obtained through the use of an amplifier.
3. Much effort was involved in playing the sixteenth notes. This seems an excessive refinement, and it is recommended that all notes should be rounded up to the nearest eighth note. If this were done, it would be possible to use paraprofessionals instead of experienced musicians.
4. No useful purpose is served by repeating with horns the passage that has already been handled by the strings. If all such redundant passages were eliminated, the concert could be reduced from two hours to twenty minutes.
5. This symphony had two movements. If Schubert didn't achieve his musical goals by the end of the first movement, then he should have stopped there.

The second movement is unnecessary and should be cut. In light of the above, one can only conclude that had Schubert given attention to these matters, he probably would have had the time to finish his symphony.
—Classic managed care joke, source unknown

How Do Medical Necessity Determinations Work?

Medical necessity determination is not a clinical decision.

The managed care company is making a decision about treatment reimbursement.

Understanding medical necessity requires, first of all, an understanding of what medical necessity isn't. *Medical necessity determination* is not a clinical decision, nor is it a clinical concept of relevance to the practice of psychotherapy, despite the name. The managed care company is making a decision about treatment reimbursement. So, at its most fundamental, medical necessity is a kind of code governing the rationing of benefits.

NCQA (2000, UM 2.4) requires that managed behavioral care companies use written criteria for the purposes of *utilization review*, which is another term for the process of looking at a client's current clinical status and the treatment plan and making a decision regarding reimbursement. The accreditation requirements also state that practitioners must be sent a copy of these utilization review criteria on request.

The document published by the managed behavioral care company that defines medical necessity for that company may be called:

- Medical Necessity Criteria (or Guidelines).
- Utilization Review Criteria (or Guidelines).
- Utilization Management Criteria (or Guidelines).
- Level of Care Criteria (or Guidelines).

Some companies routinely distribute their guidelines to professionals when they join the network; others only send them out upon telephone or written request. Larger companies, such as United Behavioral Health, Magellan, and ValueOptions, now offer a copy of the medical necessity criteria on their respective web sites (see Appendix).

The case managers use the medical necessity criteria to justify continued authorization for treatment. After reviewing the case as presented either in a telephone review or in writing, the case manager's job is to document what aspects of the patient's condition meet which section in the guidelines. The managed care company, at least in theory, expects the case manager to be able to quote chapter and verse from the company's medical necessity criteria. Treatment that fails to meet the requirements for the requested level of care is denied.

In practice, utilization management criteria are open to a good deal of interpretation, based on the specifics of the account. A managed behavioral care organization usually has only one document known as "Medical Necessity Criteria," but there are numerous accounts in both the private and public sectors. Although all case management teams use the same document, they use it differently. Despite efforts to standardize medical necessity determinations, there are two features of accounts that cause variance across teams on reimbursement decisions. The first of these two factors the therapist can find out; the second will never be revealed, because it is considered highly proprietary information:

1. The client's benefit plan.
2. The nature of the purchaser's contract with the managed care company.

Benefit Plan

Obviously, a case manager can be more generous in authorizing sessions if the client's plan allows 40 outpatient sessions per year than if it only allows 20. But that's the merest tip of the iceberg; the degree of difficulty of obtaining re-authorization is much more complex than just knowing the patient's benefit plan.

Nature of the Managed Care Contract

There are two general types of contracts. One type is called an *administrative services only* or ASO, contract. The other is called an *at-risk*, or sometimes just a *risk*, contract. The ASO contract means that the managed care company provides whatever services are requested by the employer, health plan, or government entity (utilization review, network administration, claims payment, etc.), and builds the cost of those services into its bid. In other words, the purchaser reimburses the managed care company for the treatment costs, plus a set figure for the administrative costs. The managed care company operating under an ASO contract makes the same amount of money whether it denies or authorizes treatment.

The at-risk accounts are more stereotypically managed care, and work the same way as a capitated contract (see Chapter 15). The managed care company is paid a specified amount per member per month which must cover both treatment and administration. If they authorize too much care, and spend more than they are paid, the company loses money. If there is money left over at the end of the fiscal year, that money is profit for the managed care company. Denying treatment, therefore, incurs a financial reward.

The implications for obtaining a medically necessary verdict are obvious: It's easier with an ASO account than with a risk account, even if the client has the same number of sessions allowed per year by the benefit plan. Managed care companies are also more generous in terms of the number of sessions with ASO accounts. This was consistently reported by case managers, regardless of which managed care company employed them. When asked how many sessions (or inpatient days) could be given at one time, the answer was always, "It depends on the contract." Not, as might be expected, "it depends on the benefit plan." Norman Hering recounted his company had a policy of conducting a thorough in-depth review of a client's clinical status and treatment (beyond a written treatment report) if the client had had more than a certain number of sessions authorized in one treatment episode. If the account was at-risk, clients would be reviewed after 30 sessions. However, these reviews would take place after only 50 to 60 certified sessions when the contract was ASO.

Whenever features of the patient's account/benefit plan differ from the managed behavioral care company's "Medical Necessity Guidelines," the account-specific rules will take precedence.

Whenever features of the patient's account/benefit plan differ from the managed behavioral care company's "Medical Necessity Guidelines," the account-specific rules will take precedence.

Common Features of Medical Necessity Guidelines

Every managed behavioral care company breaks down its medical necessity criteria according to level of care. Some companies then further subdivide their criteria into Mental Health, Substance Abuse, and Dual-Diagnosis. Distinct criteria for children and adolescents are also becoming a common feature in medical necessity or utilization management guidelines.

For each level of care, or subdivided level of care by type of client, there are then separate criteria for:

1. Admission.
2. Continued treatment.
3. Service (or "administrative") criteria.

Admission criteria are used to determine the initial authorization. The intake clinician at the managed care company is responsible for determining whether clients meet medical necessity standards when the call is made for precertification. It's the concurrent review or continued treatment criteria that has the most relevance to outpatient psychotherapy. Case managers reviewing outpatient treatment reports are using the continued treatment criteria from the medical necessity guidelines.

Service Components

Service components are features of the treating professional and/or setting which have nothing to do with the nature of the patient's clinical presentation, but which the managed care company nonetheless expects will be met—or treatment will not be authorized. Sometimes the medical necessity criteria document doesn't differentiate between clinical elements of medical necessity and service characteristics, but simply lists the administrative components alongside the clinical indicators. The most common service components for outpatient care are:

- An independently licensed professional (thereby excluding those under supervision).
- Face-to-face sessions (telephone or Internet sessions typically are not covered).

Sometimes there is a further restriction placed on the type of degree or license of the psychotherapist, although usually this is a restriction determined by the account rather than the managed care company as a whole. The higher levels of care must meet even more stringent administrative service characteristics. For example, intensive outpatient (IOP) and partial hospitalization programs sometimes have to be a certain number of hours per week. Facility-based programs have to be JCAHO-accredited (verified by the credentialing staff, not the case manager). Other common requirements are concerned with psychiatric coverage and supervision, availability and ratios of nurses, staff credentials, availability of certain kinds of groups and family programs, and so on.

Denials due to a professional or facility not meeting service component criteria are considered administrative rather than clinical in nature (see Chapter 12). Usually, exceptions for a failure to meet the required service components will only be made in rural areas where there are no alternative professionals or facilities to provide the care.

Case managers reviewing outpatient treatment reports are using the continued treatment criteria from the medical necessity guidelines.

The Medical Necessity Formula for Outpatient Therapy

Diagnosis and Symptoms

The major carve-out MBHOs are fairly similar in the nature of their medical necessity criteria, but the specificity of their guidelines does tend to vary, particularly for outpatient psychotherapy. The first—and universal—requirement is that there be an Axis I diagnosis (no "V" Codes accepted). Some managed behavioral care company guidelines will allow an Axis II diagnosis, but with qualifications (see Chapter 11). However, not all companies' utilization review criteria documents come right out and specify that an actual diagnosis must be given (although in practice this is what happens). They will use language such as "psychiatric symptoms," "disturbances in affect," "behavioral dysfunction," and so on. In addition to the actual diagnosis, managed care reviewers expect a verbal or written description of the symptoms which have led to the patient being given that diagnosis.

The first—and universal—requirement is that there be an Axis I diagnosis (no "V" Codes accepted).

In addition to the actual diagnosis, managed care reviewers expect a verbal or written description of the symptoms which have led to the patient being given that diagnosis.

After the Axis I Diagnosis, What Then?

Closely related to the Axis I diagnosis in the managed care mindset is the concept of *impairment in functioning*, usually in one or more life realms such as occupation, school, family, friends, financial, activities of daily living (ADLs), and so on. If one thinks about it, though, "impairment in functioning" can be somewhat vague.

> 20-year-old Teri sought therapy to address the question of whether she should seek out her biological parents. She had the typical anxieties related to this situation: worries that her adoptive parents would feel betrayed, fears that she might discover she had never been wanted, and that her biological parents would reject her overtures now, fears about the kind of people they are, and so on.

Let's say that Teri missed several of her college courses during the semester, because she was preoccupied with getting information from the state and various adoption agencies about the process of finding her birth parents. Is this an "impairment" in functioning? Would the absences in themselves suffice as impairment, or would Teri's grades have to slip? Just about anything can seem to be an impairment—if presented in accordance with the managed care way of thinking. Let's say this is a question on an outpatient treatment report:

Why is this client's treatment medically necessary?

Effective response: Teri is obsessed by the need to find her birth parents, is thinking about her search constantly, which has led to inability to concentrate on her schoolwork, and problems in educational functioning (missing classes to make calls to state and private adoption agencies, which can negatively impact her grades).

Ineffective response: Teri is obsessed by the need to find her birth parents. This is a crucial task she must undertake as she develops her adult identity.

Both statements are true, are they not? It's just that the ineffective response is not coming from the perspective that managed care has deemed the correct one.

Appropriate-Level-of-Care Standard

Most medical necessity criteria make some sort of statement to the effect that outpatient therapy must be the correct level of care. It's tied in with the whole "impairment in functioning" idea. This seems like clinical common sense: The client's functioning must be impaired, but not so greatly as to need a more intensive level of care. The managed care company is looking for things such as the presence of a family/social support system, ability to do ADLs, ability to go to work, not suicidal or homicidal, not actively abusing alcohol/drugs, and so on. It's not a hard standard to meet.

Sometimes, though, case managers do question why a client is not in a higher level of care if the client seems to be highly impaired from the case manager's perspective or if the practitioner is asking for outpatient sessions several times per week. Questions from the case manager regarding whether a client needs more intensive treatment are generally not a reflection of the case manager's opinion of the therapist's abilities. Instead, the case manager is doing his or her job. If the client's benefit plan only allows 20 outpatient sessions per year, twice weekly therapy will use a year's worth of benefits in two and a half months. Part of the case manager's job when assessing medical necessity is to consider whether another level of care would be more effective at helping the client reach the same treatment goals while conserving limited benefits.

Questions from the case manager regarding whether a client needs more intensive treatment are generally not a reflection of the case manager's opinion of the therapist's abilities.

Part of the case manager's job when assessing medical necessity is to consider whether another level of care would be more effective at helping the client reach the same treatment goals while conserving limited benefits.

Targeted Treatment Plan

*Most medical
necessity
guidelines specify
clearly that
treatment must
focus on symptom
reduction and
restoration of
functioning, or
the resolution of a
specific problem.*

Most medical necessity guidelines specify clearly that treatment must focus on symptom reduction and restoration of functioning, or the resolution of a specific problem. The medical necessity codes tend to direct, in most cases, how the therapist should work, specifying that the symptoms/problem must be resolvable with brief, solution-focused or problem-focused treatment. ValueOptions (1999), whose guidelines for outpatient treatment are highly detailed, even classifies different types of outpatient treatment and specifies goals and treatment approaches—as well as numbers of sessions—for each.

Resolvable

This is the most intangible of the medical necessity criteria. The criterion of resolvability may be expressed as, "the problem for which the client is seeking treatment is able to be resolved through outpatient psychotherapy," "the patient is motivated to make changes," and/or "there is evidence that the patient will benefit as a result of active treatment at this level of care." Sounds so obvious as to almost be a non-issue, doesn't it? Don't be fooled: This seemingly innocent little statement can be the most difficult of the "medical necessity" criteria to satisfy.

*It's the
resolvability clause
that managed care
companies tend to
use when they
think they've paid
for too many
sessions and are
looking for a way
to deny.*

Part of the problem is in measuring resolvability or benefit. As worded by the codes of medical necessity, it's certainly not a measurable standard, and it ends up being left to the case manager's interpretation. It's the resolvability clause that managed care companies tend to use when they think they've paid for too many sessions and are looking for a way to deny.

Justa Therapist, PhD, had been working with Rose Jones, age 60, for over a year, and the managed care company had authorized about 80 sessions. Rose's benefits entitled her to unlimited outpatient sessions as long as the managed care company, HPBH, certified them as "medically necessary." Rose had multiple problems, many of them medical in origin. She had had both knees operated on, and a rod inserted in her back. The orthopedic problems, causing chronic pain, were compounded by obesity, as Rose weighed about 350 pounds. She was highly resistant to engaging in exercise or maintaining herself on meal plans. Her diagnosis was Panic Disorder with Agoraphobia. Rose never left home except for therapy or doctors' appointments. She was usually highly anxious and tended to eat to calm her anxiety. There was also a significant amount of depression, anhedonia, low energy, sadness, and tearfulness. She was on medications for both the anxiety and the depression.

Except for an elderly mother who lived with her, and the nurse who came to help her mother, Rose had no social contacts. She had never married or had children.

Underneath it all, Rose had a lot of anger and rage stored away that occasionally directed itself in verbal assaults on her mother. Her father, now deceased, had been alcoholic and sexually abusive to her, and Rose had always been heavy as a way to scare off men. Her mother had been, and remained, highly critical.

Rose certainly isn't the type of client for whom "brief, solution-focused therapy" is going to do much. There are multiple problems: the anxiety, the depression, the obesity, managing the chronic pain, the over-eating, the buried rage, the relationship with her mother, the past trauma of the sexual abuse. As is so often the case in clinical "real life," all these problems tie in with one another.

Judging by all except the resolvability criterion for medical necessity, there should be no question that Rose should continue to have treatment reimbursed by HPBH. There are certainly symptoms and impairments in functioning galore, nor is Rose at such high, imminent risk to herself or others that she needs a higher level of care. But from the managed care company's point of view, where will treatment with Rose end? Although she's certainly not a short-term therapy case, neither is she severely and persistently mentally ill. At some point, the company is not going to want to continue to authorize treatment for a patient like Rose, and it's the resolvability clause in the utilization management guidelines that will enable the managed care company to find grounds for denial.

Dr. Therapist received a phone call from Kay Smanager at HPBH, notifying her that HPBH had serious concerns about whether continued therapy with Rose was likely to achieve any extra benefit. Their contention was that most of Rose's issues were lifelong concerns, and that she was doing as well as she had ever done. Furthermore, she was on medication and was being monitored by a psychiatrist, which would continue. HPBH argued that Rose could continue to maintain the same level of functioning without seeing Dr. Therapist, since she was obviously "not that motivated to lose the weight recommended by her doctor."

How long would a managed care company give a patient like Rose? It's rarely an exact number, and depends on the type of contract the managed care company has signed with the purchaser—unless the benefit plan is so limited that the patient exhausts his or her benefits first. Often, it is higher than the stereotypes would suggest (maybe even as high as 80–150 sessions), because the more sessions which have been granted, the firmer the ground for upholding an appealed denial. The following circumstances are particularly vulnerable to resolvability clauses:

- *Involuntary treatment.* Particularly in the case of adults or adolescents mandated to go through substance abuse treatment after an alcohol/drug-related offense, adolescents required to get counseling as part of a juvenile correction program, or mandated treatment for perpetrators of domestic violence or child abuse. Courts often refer these clients to private practitioners or independent facilities; in most cases, states can no longer afford to operate these types of programs. However, once involuntary status is revealed, the patient risks being denied reimbursement by managed care, unless there is "proof" that he or she is motivated. Managed care companies make the argument that involuntary treatment means a client isn't motivated, and without motivation, the treatment is not likely to lead to the client's achieving the goal(s).

- *A patient who has reached a therapeutic plateau.* While in theory this seems to be reasonable, there are many patients like Rose, the ones with numerous long-term issues but who are not severely and persistently mentally ill. These patients are doubly vulnerable to denials by making only very slow and small amounts of progress, but who are at relatively lower risk for hospitalization if their functioning deteriorates.

- *Chronic stressful situations.* Consider the classic example of a wife living with an alcoholic and/or physically abusive husband, but who has not been able to make the decision to leave. Managed care companies, particularly those with tightly managed at-risk contracts, will argue that the symptoms are a result of the situation, which can be changed, and thus can't be regarded as anything more than an Adjustment Disorder. Or, if the symptoms are severe enough, they will insist on medication, and then when the symptoms are stabilized, make this pronouncement. Patients may be expected by managed care to make do with Al-Anon or similar community support or self-help groups until they are ready to leave.

Managed care companies make the argument that involuntary treatment means a client isn't motivated, and without motivation, the treatment is not likely to lead to the client's achieving the goal(s).

- *Resolving past trauma.* Similar to chronic stressful situations, patients presenting with Post-Traumatic Stress Disorder around issues of abuse in childhood, other family of origin dysfunction, or accidents resulting in permanent physical disability, aren't likely to be authorized for their entire course of treatment. At some point, the managed care company will use the "Get Over It" argument: that past circumstances cannot be changed, and the therapist is being ineffective at producing results in a short amount of time.

Note that severe and persistent mental illness is not listed. Why not? Certainly it's not resolvable through outpatient therapy, or even by medication. Patients must manage their illnesses, engage in prevention, and take medication for the rest of their lives, but are never "cured." The advent of mental health parity laws, and the long-overdue realization that ignoring maintenance treatment leads to higher long-term hospitalization and other financial costs (not to mention human suffering), have managed to exempt severe and persistent mental illness, thankfully, from the resolvability criterion for medical necessity.

"Medical Necessity" formula for outpatient psychotherapy:

Non-clinical: Service Components

Clinical: Diagnosis + Symptoms + Impairments in Functioning + Appropriate level of care + Resolvability + Targeted treatment plan = "Medical Necessity"

Surely there's more? Not for the "medical necessity" process. There aren't any DRGs, there's no magic formula that says Major Depression gets 15 sessions, OCD gets 30, and so on. Contrary to popular perception, utilization management guidelines do not mandate psychotropic medications for certain types of patients (see Chapter 11).

But we're not out of the woods just yet. Medical necessity criteria are spawning a new breed, the highly diagnostic-specific best practices guidelines. The medical necessity determination is simply a yes or a no. The client either meets criteria, and is authorized, or does not and is denied. Even though realities such as type of contract and benefit plan factor into the equation, medical necessity is still, ultimately, a red light/green light decision. At one time, medical necessity criteria seemed invasive and directive; although many therapists still do perceive them this way, they are mild compared to the next storm brewing on the horizon, the best practices guidelines.

Unlike medical necessity criteria, best practices guidelines actually rate the effectiveness, utility, and desirability of specific treatment interventions— and are much more directive to practitioners in which methods to use for which types of patients.

Unlike medical necessity criteria, best practices guidelines actually rate the effectiveness, utility, and desirability of specific treatment interventions—and are much more directive to practitioners in which methods to use for which types of patients.

From Medical Necessity Criteria to Best Practices

There is a growing trend in the mental health field to further define and quantify what constitutes "good" and "effective" practice for each specific diagnostic issue or problem area. These *best practices guidelines*, also known as *clinical practice guidelines*, *expert consensus guidelines*, or *evidence-based treatment guidelines*, unlike medical necessity criteria, are intended to provide guidance to the practitioner in doing his or her job.

Some practice guidelines concern themselves with assessment; others with treatment. In and of themselves, guidelines may be unrelated to managed care, unless published by one of the MBHOs. The American Psychiatric Association, for example, has published guidelines on major depression, psychiatric assessment, bipolar disorder, eating disorders, panic disorder, and schizophrenia. But managed care companies are beginning to catch onto the trend, with potentially serious implications for the delivery of services over the next decade.

What Are Practice Guidelines?

Guidelines differ depending on the author of the guidelines, their purpose, and the audience for whom they are written. They range from a few pages published by a managed care company which consist of very obvious statements such as "be sure to assess for suicide risk," to hundreds of pages of scientific meta-analysis published by the APA about which antidepressant should be favored given specific medical circumstances, intended for use by psychiatrists when prescribing medication. In general, though, treatment guidelines attempt to accomplish numerous feats in one document:

1. Summarize the existing knowledge about assessment and/or treatment of a disorder.
2. Summarize the relative efficacies of the various known treatments for the disorder (including both medication and psychotherapy).
3. Provide additional continuing education for busy practitioners who don't always have time to keep up with the research literature.
4. Help practitioners consider numerous factors in making the decision regarding which treatment is most appropriate for a given patient.
5. Set a minimum standard of practice, based on research findings, which will narrow the currently wide variability in quality of assessment and treatment.

None of this, in itself, is controversial. Nobody argues with the fact that the mental health field as a whole has a lot of work yet to do with regard to defining and measuring outcomes and effectiveness. The overwhelming majority of clinicians would agree that the above goals are admirable. But as the managed care companies get involved, practice guidelines become a highly controversial issue.

Developing Clinical Practice Guidelines: A Function of Managed Care Companies?

Bea Worker, case manager at GenRUs Behavioral Health, went to a mandatory training conducted by the Clinical Director of her unit. The CD unveiled the new *GBH PPP: Preferred Practice Patterns*, meant to supplement the Utilization Management Guidelines. It was developed using GBH's database of several million cases.

"No one else," said the CD, "is in the same unique position as GBH to advance the science of quantifiable, evidence-based treatment. Certainly not our providers, who have access only to their small numbers of cases. Each provider might see only one or two eating disorders a year, for example. But now, with GBH's PPP in hand, the providers have at their fingertips a wealth of knowledge gleaned from thousands of cases across the country."

There are serious concerns about the quality of practice guidelines that are developed on a strictly in-house basis, where the managed care company owns the outcome, and where the development process is protected by the veil of proprietary information.

Number-Crunching

First, top-level management chooses a clinical area for development of the best practices guidelines. Once a diagnostic category or problem is chosen, there are two statistical methods possible for managed care companies to use to go about formulating their treatment guidelines. One way, an internal-data approach, described to me by a statistical analyst employed at one of the Top 5, is to analyze several years' worth of accumulated data from clinical and claims records, and from satisfaction/outcome measures, on all patients with a given diagnosis.

The other method is to use an outside consulting firm for the statistical analysis. Milliman & Robertson, in Seattle, sell "Healthcare Management Guidelines" which are actuarially-derived analyses from utilization data sold to them by managed care companies (Miller, 1999). Smaller companies, in particular, prefer this method because they can thus buy a larger sample. If depression, for example, is treated in roughly 10 percent of a company's "covered lives," but there are only a half-million "covered lives," then sample size is a concern.

Whether the numbers remain in-house or are obtained from Milliman & Robertson or a similar type of company is actually irrelevant for the purposes of judging the quality of the final practice guidelines (although there are antitrust concerns that arise from the latter approach), because both methods have serious, obvious flaws. As Ivan Miller points out, ". . . standards cannot be set by looking at utilization rates alone. Differences in practice patterns can represent patterns of undertreatment as well as overtreatment. The clear presumption in the Milliman & Robertson literature is that if there is a difference in length of treatment or treatment rates between populations the more expensive treatment must be a result of inefficiencies."

Remember the Control Group?

Anyone who remembers this most basic of concepts from Research Methods 101 in grad school can identify the fundamental concern about making conclusions about effectiveness of various treatments based on statistical methods alone. There's no control group. Where is an adequately-sized sample of clients who have the same diagnosis but who have received alternative treatments? Managed care openly reinforces certain kinds of treatment through financial reimbursement, and penalizes other types through the threat or actual withdrawal of financial assistance to the therapy process. So the managed care data sample is inherently skewed toward patients who are already receiving brief, solution-focused treatment, which, moreover, is subject to periodic medical necessity review by case managers. From the statistical analyses, how can any sort of meaningful conclusion be made about relative effectiveness of various treatments when there is really only one—the shortest possible—which is being studied?

This is not to say that managed care shouldn't be involved in best practices development. The managed care companies' contribution is access to a vast sample size, more than hitherto ever possible. But statistical analysis in and of itself is not the whole answer.

What's the Big Secret?   Because managed care clearly stands to gain economically from practice guidelines which recommend ultra-brief and psychopharmacological treatment, the development of proprietary best practices guidelines behind closed doors will almost surely lead to widespread practitioner skepticism of the guidelines' clinical utility.

Ivan Miller (1999) has formulated standards for guideline development:

1. A thorough report of the procedure and process of deliberation of treatment guideline panels must be open to public review.
2. The identity, interests, and qualifications of the members of a guideline panel must be open to public and professional review.
3. The guidelines panel must clearly identify restrictions on the patients' conditions, type of mental health care professional, settings, and goals.
4. The guideline panel must fully report its rationale for each guideline, and separately report the rationale for each conceptually distinct goal such as cost, effectiveness, ethical, and legal considerations.
5. Guideline panels must design a method of evaluating, correcting, and revising treatment guidelines.
6. Complete treatment guidelines, including financial incentives, rules, recommendations, policies, or other means of guiding the delivery of treatment services, must be fully described with appropriate statistics and accompanying data in order that all of the factors that function as guidelines can be scrutinized by professionals, scientists, and consumer advocates.

From the statistical analyses, how can any sort of meaningful conclusion be made about relative effectiveness of various treatments when there is really only one—the shortest possible—which is being studied?

Alternatives: The Collaborative Approach to Practice Guideline Development

The professional and mental health advocacy literature is overwhelmingly in support of nonproprietary, professional development of practice guidelines (e.g., Pomerantz, 1999a). There are already single-discipline guidelines out there, such as the ones developed and published by both APA's, the American Society of Addiction Medicine (ASAM), and the American Academy of Child and Adolescent Psychiatry, among others. In fact, the Agency for Healthcare Policy and Research, a division of the U.S. Department of Health and Human Services, sponsors an Internet-based National Guideline Clearinghouse, which catalogs and describes medical and behavioral health guidelines—including the process of the guidelines' development (see Appendix).

Could it actually be beginning? There is also a multidisciplinary initiative, with numerous professional organizations participating, known as the Practice Guidelines Coalition or PGC (see Appendix).

"What does all this have to do with my private practice?" It's so tempting to assume that all this is political maneuvering and posturing without relevance to everyday practice. But best practices guidelines are already beginning to affect the authorization of treatment, and hold serious implications, legitimized by NCQA, for *provider profiling*.

Implementing Best Practices Guidelines in Approving Treatment

Should therapists be accountable for outcomes or interventions? Even with the most impeccable of guideline development processes, though, the mere fact that clinicians are to be held accountable for the choice of clinical interventions, rather than for outcomes, is a bit disturbing. It's clear from their name that best practices guidelines focus on "how:" how to assess, how to treat.

To the managed care way of thinking, if we can demonstrate that for problem Y, Intervention A is equally or more clinically effective than Interventions B or C, but Intervention A is the least costly of the three alternatives, then doesn't it make sense to use Intervention A as the first-choice treatment strategy? Leaving aside the fact that mental health/ substance abuse interventions are rarely so clear-cut, there are other concerns with the implementation of practice guidelines by managed care:

1. The philosophy clashes with the value of free choice by the patient, in conjunction with his or her therapist.
2. Practitioners are, naturally, going to perceive directives from managed care to use Intervention A as being directive of treatment in order to increase profits.
3. Although this might be considered acceptable treatment rationing where resources are scarce and there is a single-payer health care system, in the American health care system there are profits being made which take resources away from treatment.
4. Can such policy decisions ethically be made in the absence of studies that document the long-term effects of various interventions? Intervention A may be demonstrated to produce good immediate outcomes, but is it as good or better than Interventions B and C in the long term at preventing relapse/decompensation?
5. Who should define the minimum "acceptable" level of quality, now that this function is removed from the traditional joint effort by the practitioner and patient? Employers? The government? Or managed care, which has a clear economic incentive under at-risk contracts?

Lest anyone think this mere alarmist talk, #5, for instance, is already being played out in the *fail-first* policies implemented by the drug formularies of various HMOs. In an effort to control the costs of prescription medications, newer and more expensive antipsychotic drugs such as Risperidone and Olanzapine are often denied unless the patient clearly "fails" on an older, cheaper drug, usually with more side effects, such as Haldol. But what is "failure?" If the Haldol controls the psychosis but leaves the patient feeling like a zombie, causes unpleasant dry mouth and a few hand tremors, is that "success" or "failure?"

Reimbursement of Psychotherapy in Private Practice

Justa Therapist, PhD, read the latest missive from GenRUs Behavioral Health in horror:

Dear Participating Provider

GenRUs Behavioral Health proudly unveils its Preferred Practice Patterns which will standardize treatment available to all members and raise the bar on quality. In accordance with the standards of the National Committee for Quality Assurance, GBH will periodically monitor provider adherence to these guidelines to ensure the highest possible quality of care for our members.

One GBH PPP guideline outlined the circumstances under which patients were to be referred for antidepressant medication:

1. Symptoms lasting longer than 2 months;
2. Concurrent anxiety;
3. If more than 2 days of work have been missed in the last month;
4. Within 3 weeks of beginning treatment for any patient with a previous history of depression, treated or untreated;
5. The patient must be referred to a psychiatrist on the GBH panel, not a primary care physician.

Companies that implement formal treatment guidelines have a responsibility to communicate what the explicit reimbursement consequences will be for the patient if a decision is made to deviate from the guidelines.

What this may mean to Dr. Therapist in practice with clients is that reimbursement for treatment may be denied or reduced unless she honors the "rules" as set forth in GBH's Preferred Practice Patterns. Companies that implement formal treatment guidelines have a responsibility to communicate what the explicit reimbursement consequences will be for the patient if a decision is made to deviate from the guidelines. To date, this is not happening, nor is it mandated to do so by NCQA's (2000) QI 7 standard, which addresses the implementation of "best practices" guidelines.

Having to be accountable to a guideline also underscores the importance of an open guideline development process. Practitioners need meaningful reassurance that the guideline is truly an exercise in raising the standard of quality rather than in raising the profit margin. If GBH includes detailed information, such as the relevant statistics, citations from the professional research literature, and a description of the guideline development process, Dr. Therapist could educate herself as to the clinical appropriateness of the guideline, and would thus be more likely to adhere to it, assuming it was clinically sound.

Setting the Standard

Pomerantz (1999a) argues that practice guidelines, if done right, set a minimum standard of care that can be used to more realistically define malpractice in the age of managed care. If Pomerantz is right, then the importance of practice guidelines to each therapist cannot be understated, as the guidelines which are adopted will irrevocably alter the standard of care from a legal standpoint. But what if the guidelines are created using a distorted and proprietary statistical process, by companies whose primary motive is to preserve profits? If Dr. Therapist, for example, should ever face a lawsuit, how could she successfully answer a charge of malpractice if she did not refer a patient for medications, according to the guideline issued by GBH? The danger is that the managed care companies, by virtue of sheer size and economic influence, might someday be able to determine prevailing standards of practice—even for professionals who choose not to participate on the networks.

Best Practices Guidelines in Provider-Profiling

NCQA's accreditation *Standards* say quite plainly that "the organization annually measures adherence to at least two of the guidelines" (NCQA, 2000, QI 7.5). NCQA also specifies that the MBHOs must put in place a system to monitor exceptions from the guidelines (NCQA, 2000, QI 7.6).

There are potential dangers to measuring adherence to best practices guidelines. What about legitimate clinical differences of opinion? This is not necessarily a sign of "managed care unfriendliness." Nor does it seem feasible to have to obtain an exception from the managed care company in the event of such disagreement. Will clinicians who economically depend on managed care really be able to make appropriate recommendations to their clients, if they know that they are expected to practice a certain way, and that the conformity of their practice to the guidelines is being monitored? Or will it result in what Miller (1996) calls a "covert gag," and operate like a contractual gag clause, where the therapist simply does not inform the patient of more expensive or noncovered treatment options?

The danger is that the managed care companies, by virtue of sheer size and economic influence, might someday be able to determine prevailing standards of practice—even for professionals who choose not to participate on the networks.

8

Requesting Additional Sessions

Dina Troy, LCSW, is reviewing her charts for the next day's sessions. She opens the file for UCBH client Judy Schmoe and realizes there's no current certification letter. But she's positive she sent a treatment report for reauthorization at least a month, maybe even 6 weeks ago. What happened?

When Dina called to inquire, the Customer Service rep said "I'm sorry, we show no record of receiving it. You'll need to send it again, and none of the sessions held without authorization will be paid."

What could have happened to Dina's outpatient treatment report (OTR), the written request for additional sessions that contains updated clinical information? Just about anything. She may have inadvertently sent it to the wrong UCBH fax number or post office box, or it could have fallen into a "black hole," once arrived at the company.

Why Do "Black Holes" Exist?

Each account team at the large managed behavioral care carve-out firms receive hundreds of reports daily. Even if the company maintains a database of each and every report received, the odds are that some items will still get lost. All the little things that can go wrong, do, sometimes. Fax machines run out of paper and toner cartridge, and the memory fills up. The person taking the faxes off the machine drops a sheet or somehow doesn't get all the pages together. Mail and faxes can be mis-routed or simply lost, and so on.

Managed care companies should make a decision about continued certification for outpatient treatment within 2 weeks (10 working days).

Because of the black-hole phenomenon, it's in a therapist's best interest to call the managed care company to verify receipt and review of the OTR before too much time has gone by. How long to wait after sending the report? Per NCQA (2000), Standard UM 4.1.7.2, managed care companies should make a decision about continued certification for outpatient treatment within 2 weeks (10 working days). But therapists may not even have to wait that long. Performance guarantees promising faster turnaround times for outpatient treatment reports than the NCQA standard (often as few as 5 working days) are commonplace.

Follow-Up Etiquette and Documentation

The numbers tell the entire story of why follow-up is so absolutely vital. If a therapist is seeing a client weekly, and sends an OTR requesting 8 sessions, it can take up to 2 weeks to be reviewed, and may then be another 2 weeks before the authorization letter is received at the therapist's office. The therapist might easily have used 4 sessions of an 8-session authorization before actually obtaining proof of authorization. Table 8.1 summarizes the major ways in which therapists can protect themselves against claims denials due to "lost" OTRs.

When following up, don't ask to speak to the case manager. Unless there is a clinical question in tandem with a request for verification of receipt, don't bother a clinician. They're there to review OTRs, not go hunting

Unless there is a clinical question in tandem with a request for verification of receipt, don't bother a clinician.

Table 8.1
Ten Steps to Obtaining Recertification

1. When verifying benefits and/or pre-authorizing, make it a matter of routine to obtain the address for OTRs.
2. Always do the treatment plan 2 to 3 weeks before the last certified session to allow for receipt and review of the OTR by the time the client needs the first session of the new authorization.
3. Keep a copy of every OTR sent in the client's file, along with proof of receipt: either the fax transmission report, or the green certified return receipt card issued by the Post Office.
4. If faxing, use a cover page indicating how many pages are in the transmission, and a telephone number to contact in the event not all the pages are received. Clearly number the pages and make sure the client's name and/or ID number appears on every page.
5. Call in 2 to 3 weeks to follow up that the OTR was received and reviewed—before the first unauthorized session takes place.
6. Minimize the time spent on follow up calls by asking about several patients at once wherever possible.
7. Get the name and extension of the person you talk to and keep with the copy of the OTR, along with a notation of the date the follow-up call was made and what you were told. This information may be critical later, if claims end up denied.
8. Be sure to ask for a certification/authorization number.
9. Be sure to inquire not only what is the number of sessions authorized, but also about the start and end dates and the type of session/CPT code authorized.
10. Request a printed certification letter if one has not yet been received.

for them. Instead, use customer service; reps can give out authorization information on the phone. Customer service reps are expected to document who is calling, for what purpose, and what is told to them—a fact that can be used to the therapist's advantage if there is a problem with receipt of an OTR.

Never leave a voice mail for following up receipt/review of an OTR. The recipient of the voice mail must search for the OTR, wait for the computer to pull up the client's file, call the therapist back, and make a note summarizing the action taken. Calling to say, "the OTR is on its way" is the same trap, because voice mails or live calls of this sort have a high likelihood of not getting documented. And anything that's not documented didn't happen.

Are they truly that overworked? Yes. Outpatient case managers typically have a caseload of 1,500 to 2,000 names. If they get 10 calls or voice mails of this sort each day, at 5 minutes each that's almost an hour of an 8-hour day used; at 10 minutes each that's more than an hour and a half. Outpatient case managers have a quota of treatment reports to do each day, and it's usually set fairly high to allow the turnaround standards to be met. Customer service reps must take a quota of calls each day (see Chapter 1).

Should I cancel/reschedule the next appointment if the company claims they didn't receive the OTR? Not recommended. If the client needs to be treated, but isn't seen because of screw-ups with the managed care company authorization process, and something then happens to the client, who is more likely to be seen as legally negligent—the therapist or the managed care company? More everyday ramifications of canceling a client's appointment due to authorization problems are likely to be client complaints, clients abandoning treatment prematurely, and the eventual tarnishing of a good professional reputation, in the community as well as at the managed care company.

An authorization for sessions that have already happened is known as a retrocertification, or back-certification, and is typically prohibited by managed care companies, where the custom is generally to begin the new authorization on the day the OTR is received.

When to Request a Retrocertification—and How to Do It Effectively

An authorization for sessions that have already happened is known as a retrocertification, or backcertification, and is typically prohibited by managed care companies, where the custom is generally to begin the new authorization on the day the OTR is received. In Dina's case, what this means is that even though she says she sent Judy's OTR a month ago,

UCBH most likely will start the new authorization only when they receive the resubmitted treatment report, and the claims for Judy's last 4 to 6 sessions will be denied.

Prove them wrong. Most companies will back-certify if the therapist can produce proof that the OTR was originally sent—and received—on a date prior to the first noncertified session. Proof usually means either a fax transmission sheet showing the correct fax number, a successful transmission, and the date, or a postal return receipt. Is it worth the extra hassle? Do the math. Is one session, even at an admittedly cut-rate fee of $45 to $65 per session, worth the two or three dollars extra (and the time) it costs to mail the OTR certified return receipt? That's an individual judgment call.

Most companies will back-certify if the therapist can produce proof that the OTR was originally sent— and received—on a date prior to the first noncertified session.

Other "Legitimate" Reasons to Grant a Retrocertification

There is usually only one: some failure on the part of the managed care company—if it can be proven by the therapist.

> Mary Caring, LCSW, sent an OTR to GenRUs Behavioral Health on 4/15/99. Two weeks later it was returned to her, marked "Incorrect Health Plan ID." Sure enough, the Health Plan ID differed by one digit from the patient's social security number. However, both numbers had been listed on the OTR. Mary checked the original authorization, which also listed both numbers, and found the same one-digit discrepancy between the two ID numbers. After calling the patient to verify the correct number, Mary sent the OTR again on 5/1/99 with a corrected "Health Plan ID" and called GBH back on 5/5/99 to request a backcertification to 4/15. Mary's request was granted.

Is this a "legitimate" reason for a retrocertification? Absolutely. For one thing, the managed care company made a typo on the authorization letter. And for another, since both numbers were shown on the original report and one was correct, the OTR could have been reviewed the first time around.

The 10 Most Common Excuses That Will Not Get a Retrocertification

Therapists requesting retrocertifications are sometimes told that "I'd help you if I could, but the computer won't let me change the date." Most often, this is usually a lie, told for reasons of self-preservation. Nobody likes to be yelled at, however, employees have to have the electronic flexibility to change authorization dates in those situations in which the managed care company deems it "valid" for them to do so. Unless a therapist who calls is lucky enough to get a disgruntled or independent-minded employee, customer service reps and case managers will play by the rules and not use their electronic capability to roll back the date on an authorization. They too have mortgages to pay and children to feed, and won't risk their jobs, no matter how sympathetic they might be.

The following excuses are heard on a daily basis, and they don't work. Don't even waste time calling; follow the advice given on what to do instead.

1. *"I haven't seen the client long enough to be able to fill one of those things out."*

   Managed Care Employee Response: "Fill it in as best you can."

   What to Do Instead: Fill it out, and consult Chapters 9 and 10 for tips. It's also very legitimate to write a note on the OTR to the effect that the patient has only been seen once, twice, etc.

2. *"I didn't fill out the OTR because I hadn't seen the client in a long time, and so I didn't know what was going on with him or her."*

   Managed Care Employee Response: "Why didn't you call before the client came back to find out what you needed to do?"

   What to Do Instead: If a client returns to treatment after the authorization has expired, always call first, just as if the client were new. Or, if the authorization has no end date, but the client hasn't been seen in a period of 90 days or longer, call. It can only go one of two ways.

   A. The case manager/customer service rep can authorize one or more sessions to re-assess the client before making the treatment plan due.

   B. They will tell you to send in a treatment plan immediately. If this is what happens, then just do it, making sure to note the gap in treatment as a reason for clinical uncertainty.

3. *"There's been no change since the last time I sent a treatment report."* (This is the worst thing a therapist can say to a case manager.)

   Care Manager Response: Why hasn't the client made progress since the last report? Is it that the client has reached a plateau and isn't

It's legitimate to write a note on the OTR to the effect that the patient has only been seen once, twice, etc.

If a client returns to treatment after the authorization has expired, always call first, just as if the client were new.

likely to achieve any further benefit from outpatient therapy? Or are you really conducting long-term exploratory or growth therapy? Either way, it's not medically necessary. Suddenly, not only the request for a retrocertification is denied, but the request for future sessions is in jeopardy.

What to Do Instead: Do the treatment plan. Surely there must be some improvement, no matter how small, even with the most resistant, chronic, or relapse-prone of patients. The trick is in identifying the progress (see Chapter 10).

4. *"You guys make it so confusing, there's no way I can keep up."* (Variation: "I can't afford office staff because you guys don't pay enough.")

   Managed Care Employee Response: While the employee might be a sympathetic audience, complaining about the state of affairs in modern American healthcare service delivery doesn't give the employee the justification he or she needs to be able to back-certify.

   What to Do Instead: Adopt a strategy to stay current. It doesn't matter what the strategy is, as long as it's reliable and works. Or, hire someone to manage managed-care tasks. Or, decide for once and for all to tear up all managed-care contracts and make a living taking only self-pay clients.

5. *"I didn't have a copy of the right form."* (Variation: "I didn't know which form to use.")

   Managed Care Employee Response: Why didn't you make a copy of the form that came with the first authorization? Or, Why didn't you call and ask which form to use and/or to be sent a form?

   What to Do Instead: Always make a copy of the blank form that arrives with the initial authorization letter, and keep the copy in the client's chart.

   Always make a copy of the blank form that arrives with the initial authorization letter, and keep the copy in the client's chart.

As a last resort, call and ask that a blank form be mailed or faxed, or ask which form to use.

Pick a Form, any Form

With all the mergers, revisions, regional- and account-specific OTR forms out there, knowing which form to use is a legitimate concern; but not sending something because of uncertainty isn't considered grounds for a retro-certification.

However, therapists who send the wrong form should at least get credit for having sent something. There have even been therapists who wrote their OTRs on a completely different company's form. As a case manager, my colleagues and I usually accepted whatever was received, then sent the correct form to the therapist with a note indicating "use this next time." Other case managers who were interviewed stated their procedures were similar. About the worst thing that should happen if a wrong form is submitted is that the therapist will receive a call from the case manager, asking for additional clinical information. Reassuringly, I've never heard of anyone being denied sessions on the basis of the wrong form being sent, or that anyone was made to do the same treatment plan over on the right form.

But it might get worse. Two trends are making it more unlikely that the "we'll accept anything" attitude will continue. The first is the increased use of computers to scan the treatment report forms, since a wrong form will, obviously, not be able to be computer-scored. The second is the use of nonclinician assistants to prescreen OTRs. Nonclinicians are likely to be more inflexible since they will have been trained to the specific company's form. In either case, one would hope that the MBHO would send the wrong form to a case manager for "live" review, rather than asking the therapist to re-do the treatment plan. But don't count on it.

6. *"You never sent the authorization letter, so I didn't know it was time."*

   Managed Care Employee Response: Why didn't you call about not getting an authorization letter?

   What to Do Instead: Find a system of tracking authorizations and treatment plans that works, and stick to it. Managed care companies do not consider it their responsibility to inform each and every therapist when they should re-submit treatment plans. And why would they? "Late" OTRs mean that they can deny claims.

7. *"There were still sessions left on the authorization"* (for companies which give a certification end date).

   Managed Care Employee Response: Why didn't you call to request an end date extension?

   What to Do Instead: Always be aware of end dates and call ahead of time to get them extended. Most of the time, the customer service rep will simply change the "good through" date and reprint the authorization.

"What if they won't extend the end date?" Some companies, unable to handle the high volume of "could you please extend the end date?" calls, have decreed that when the authorization expires, a new treatment plan must be sent, even if there are still unused sessions. The only defense against losing a session's payment to this maneuver is to be aware of end dates. Call to request a time extension enough in advance such that if they refuse, there is time to get a new treatment report in before the client's first session after the "good through" date.

Call to request a time extension enough in advance such that if they refuse, there is time to get a new treatment report in before the client's first session after the "good through" date.

Their Mistake

Maybe it's because case managers don't always count correctly. Or maybe it's a sneaky gambit to try to retain more profit. For whatever reason, every once in a while there are 8 sessions authorized at a frequency of once per week, and then only a 6-week time span allowed on the authorization. Call to point this out and request an end date extension, ideally as soon as you notice the discrepancy. Even if there's a "no end date extension" policy, such a mistake is good grounds for an exception.

As a last straw, if a session does inadvertently fall outside the certification dates, there is a good argument to use in an appeal letter, if a request for an end date extension is denied. It doesn't matter whether the "good through" date was passed because of vacation or illness on the part of either the therapist or the client, because the case manager couldn't count, or because the therapist was simply not mindful that the date had passed.

Write a letter of appeal, addressed to the Clinical Director of the particular case management team (Figure 8.1). Use a straightforward clinical argument such as the one used in the letter. Dr. Therapist might seem to be laying it on a bit thick, but her letter is likely to gain attention for the following reasons:

1. She uses a clinical argument, establishing medical necessity for the denied session.
2. She demonstrates effective clinical outcomes.
3. She uses a friendly, collaborative tone.
4. She asks for clarification of the reasons for the policy, as well as asking for the session to be reimbursed.
5. She takes responsibility for not having been aware of the end date, but also makes it clear that there was an abrupt change in policy without her having been notified.

Figure 8.1
Request for Retrocertification

July 6, 2000

Bob Bigwig II, Ph.D., Clinical Director
GenRUs Behavioral Health, Widget Company Unit
12345 Corporate Square Park
St. Louis, MO 63105

RE: John Doe, Social Security # 999-99-9999
Date of service: 5/12/2000

Dear Dr. Bigwig,

I am writing about a disturbing development, in the hopes that this matter can be resolved quickly and effectively. I have been a provider with GenRUs Behavioral Health for three years now, and to date have enjoyed good working relationships with your case managers. My record of quality treatment and high client satisfaction ratings have brought me many GBH referrals.

John Doe, a Widget Company employee, sought treatment in late January, 2000, for Major Depression. He was missing work several days out of every month. Symptoms were initial insomnia, AM hypersomnia with difficulty getting out of bed, irritability, lack of appetite, weight loss, and frequent headaches. At admission his score on the Beck Depression Inventory was a 40.

By the first part of May, John was doing significantly better. After 12 sessions, he was reporting reduced symptoms in all areas and had a BDI score of 18. As a result, we had cut back the frequency of our sessions to twice monthly, to begin the process of therapeutic termination and with the twin goals of helping John to maintain his gains, and generalize the new skills he has learned through therapy to other life situations.

On May 11, 1999, I noticed that although I had only used 6 of 8 sessions on my authorization, #RCP8594ZS1, the authorization had expired May 3rd. I called to extend the end date and was told by a Carla J. in Customer Service that GBH no longer extends end dates. I immediately sent another treatment plan, but apparently this was not received in time for the session on May 12th to be authorized.

Please help me understand the reasons for this new policy. Not extending end dates seems to be in direct contradiction to GBH's core clinical mission of cost-effective psychotherapy. Patients can consolidate their gains through additional homework during a "termination phase" of treatment where they are seen less frequently, thus reducing the risk of expensive relapses. Perhaps when formulating this policy, GBH did not consider the unintended consequence for therapists who are providing high-quality, cost-effective brief treatment.

I certainly realize that had I checked the authorization end date earlier, I would have had more time to get in a new treatment plan. However, in the past your staff has been so courteous and efficient, it certainly never occurred to me that they would refuse something so trivial as to extend an authorization "good through" date. Enclosed, please find a copy of the treatment plan originally mailed on May 11th.

Dr. Bigwig, I would ask that you rectify the matter of the denied session for May 12th. As you can see, treatment for Mr. Doe on this date was clearly medically necessary. In order to continue to provide such high quality care, and to work in partnership with GBH for the greater benefit of the Widget Company employees and their families, I must be able to cover the expenses involved in operating a practice.

Thank you very much for your consideration of this matter. I look forward to hearing from you and will certainly make myself available for any further questions which you might have.

Sincerely,

Justa Therapist, Ph.D.

Want to make the managed care company sweat a bit? If you don't mind taking the risk of tarnishing your "provider profile," and if the client gives permission, state that a copy of this letter is being sent to the benefit administrator at the client's employer. Use verbiage like this: "as a therapist truly concerned about the quality of services being offered to employees and families of [company name], I feel it is important that [company] needs to be informed as to the policies of its managed behavioral care vendor. Policies such as refusal to extend end dates negatively impact on the ability of therapists to operate practices which provide quality care in these tight economic conditions."

A bit over the top, just for a refusal to extend an end date? Yes. That's exactly the point. A letter like this usually works because the potential for negative PR is worse than paying the therapist for the denied session(s). Dr. Therapist's letter also serves as a good example of how to request a retrocertification, discussed next.

8. *"My secretary forgot to tell me."* (Variations: "My computer program didn't work," "my computer is in the shop," "my secretary was on vacation," "I have new office staff," "I was on vacation," etc.)

   Managed Care Employee Response: What can the employee say? He or she may be sympathetic, but unless he or she is willing to go out on a limb for that sympathy, there won't be a back-cert granted.

   What to Do Instead: Life happens. It's the private practitioner's responsibility to decide if "life" is happening too often and make changes to practice management systems.

9. *"The client didn't tell me I had to do this."*

   Managed Care Employee Response: [to a participating therapist] It's not the client's responsibility, it's yours. Read your contract.

   Managed Care Employee Response: [to an out-of-network therapist] When the client said he or she wanted to use insurance, why didn't you call to verify the benefits and find out what procedures to follow?

   What to Do Instead: Read that contract again. All managed-care contracts place the burden of obtaining concurrent authorization on the participating practitioner. In the case of being out-of-network, it's always best to call as soon as possible to verify benefits, obtain information about co-payments, limits, where to send the claims—and to determine if the utilization review is "managed."

10. *"The doctor just doesn't understand the need to fill these things out right away."* [from a secretary, billing person, or office manager:]

All managed-care contracts place the burden of obtaining concurrent authorization on the participating practitioner.

Managed care employees perceive rude office staff as a negative reflection on the practitioner.

Managed Care Employee Response: There's not much a managed care employee can say in response, nor is it a reason in their eyes to grant a back-certification.

What to Do Instead: If you're the secretary, billing person, or office manager, remember that you represent the doctor to the managed care company. Managed care employees perceive rude office staff as a negative reflection on the practitioner.

Requesting a Retrocertification

Make the request in a separate letter; don't simply write a note on the treatment report, as it's likely to be overlooked.

Make the request in a separate letter; *don't simply write a note on the treatment report,* as it's likely to be overlooked. Or, the case manager or clerk reviewing the OTR might not have any authority to say yes. Instead, make whatever calls are needed to discover the name and title of someone high enough up who will have the authority to grant the request.

In writing the letter, show off the quality of work that has been done with the client (Figure 8.1). Attach copies of whatever proofs are relevant, and state the case clearly. Make sure the letter is friendly in tone. Don't make excuses; if you've made mistakes, admit them, but show why it's in the best interests of the managed care company to grant the request.

Survival Tip: In a letter protesting policies or making administrative requests, never make threats, warnings, or ominous predictions that the client will clinically decompensate or relapse. There's a high risk this strategy will backfire. Managed care clinician-employees, regardless of their level in the hierarchy, may misinterpret the letter to mean that the therapist will act out and destructively triangulate the client, if the request is denied.

How Many Sessions and How Much Time?

Some companies' OTR forms don't allow the practitioner to request a specific number of sessions. And even if the forms do allow it, the company generally has an internal directive limiting the number of sessions that case managers are allowed to authorize at any one time. This number can vary widely. HMO plans which typically allow only 20 or 30 sessions per year, often review as frequently as every 4 sessions, whereas there are some companies that will authorize as many as 10 or 12 sessions at one time before requiring another OTR. Type of contract (ASO vs. at-risk) also influences the determination of maximum number of sessions per authorization (see Chapter 7).

Not Just the Managed Care Company

Influential employers, insurance plans, or other corporate/government customers can over-ride whatever the company has determined will be the maximum number of sessions for any one authorization period. The purchaser may specify either a more generous, or a more stingy maximum. I remember one client, covered by a large national managed care company that typically authorized 10 sessions at one time. This client had a fairly severe bipolar disorder, and had been recently hospitalized, but was only given 5 outpatient sessions. The medical necessity was not the issue. However, said the case manager disgustedly, when I called to ask about the short authorization periods, this client's employer specifically insisted that no more than 5 sessions be given at any one time.

The company generally has an internal directive limiting the number of sessions that case managers are allowed to authorize at any one time.

These policies have to do with the way accounts are sold, according to a former program director of a large national account at one of the Top 5 managed care companies. This program director, who asked not to be named, commented that "Sales sells what they think the customer wants. They aren't clinicians, and they sell 100 percent case management because it sounds good, even though it would be smarter fiscally just to manage the outliers." Employers may then dictate the maximum number of sessions per authorization, according to this program director, in a perceived attempt to maximize the "value-added" features offered by the company managing the care.

Sales sells what they think the customer wants. They aren't clinicians, and they sell 100 percent case management because it sounds good, even though it would be smarter fiscally just to manage the outliers.

"Hard" or "Soft?"

Managed care employees describe accounts in terms of *soft-certing* (or *easy-certing*) versus *hard-certing*. A *soft-cert* account is one in which it is relatively easy to demonstrate medical necessity and is generous in terms of the maximum number of sessions that can be given. A *hard-cert* account means that the managed care company is tighter with sessions and is more stringent with regard to determinations of "medical necessity," regardless of who originates the *hard-cert* policy.

Always find out first the maximum number of sessions the benefit plan allows. If the client has run out of benefits, no sessions will be authorized, no matter how clinically sharp an OTR, or how behavioral the treatment goals. In general, assume that the smaller the maximum session limit, the harder it will be to demonstrate medical necessity/obtain re-authorization.

"How many sessions do I ask for if I am allowed to make a request?" Table 8.2 offers general guidelines. However, watch for patterns in authorizations; if a particular company routinely authorizes a small number of sessions for clients with one specific benefit plan, it's probably due to a *hard-cert* internal policy.

Who Reviews the OTRs?

When I was a case manager, therapists were often pleasantly surprised to find out that I was a licensed clinician. Practitioners of all disciplines

Table 8.2
General Guidelines for the Number of Sessions/Amount of Time to Request

Master's and Doctoral Level Clinicians, and Psychiatrists requesting full 45–50 minute therapy sessions (with or without medication management):

- No more than 8 or 10 sessions at one time.
- No longer than 3 or 4 months at one time (if being seen weekly).
- Frequency no more than once weekly.

Psychiatrists requesting medication management for 15-minute or 30-minute sessions. (What case managers view as excessive will depend on the requested frequency of visits):

Twice monthly:

- No more than 8 or 10 sessions at one time.
- No longer than 6–8 months at one time.

Once monthly:

- No more than 6 or 8 sessions at one time.
- No longer than 9 months at one time.

Every other month or less frequently:

- No more than 4–6 sessions at one time.
- No longer than 12 months at one time.

Note: This is not to be interpreted that managed care will never authorize more. These parameters as intended only as general guidelines to avoid making requests that may be considered "excessive" or trigger a more focused review.

and license levels would admit, somewhat abashed, that "I had no idea a real clinician looks at these!"

Do clinicians always review the OTRs? Unfortunately, no. There is some truth to the rumors. Because of the heavy volume of treatment reports received by the managed care companies, it's cheaper to pay associates with a bachelor's degree, or unlicensed master's degree, to handle the majority of the load (or to have a computer do it), than it is to pay fully-licensed, experienced clinicians. Under this system, the complex reports and/or the ones in which there is a question of denial, are weeded out and sent to a licensed clinician for review. Micromanaging outpatient treatment is inherently cost-ineffective.

Micromanaging outpatient treatment is inherently cost-ineffective.

What's worse: a computer or a clerk? Computers violate confidentiality only when too many people are allowed access—or when they are hacked into. The problems with use of nonclinical staff are in the area of confidentiality rather than the risk of an inappropriate denial (see Chapter 12). Hering (1999) points out that while clinicians are trained to use supervisory or peer support to cope with disturbing clinical information, there is no such support available to the legions of nonclinical assistants and data entry clerks.

How do nonclinician managed care employees (*or computers*) know when to pass the OTR on to a clinical case manager? They are given instructions regarding what to look for. One case manager reported that in her division, there was a screening committee of assistants who initially examined the OTRs. They would select out the ones that needed review by a case manager, then certify the rest. When computers are used, any scannable OTR that doesn't pass the computer's algorithms gets sent to the case manager, who then calls the therapist for additional information and/or a telephone review, as needed.

The 10 Most Common Reasons a Treatment Report Gets a Closer Examination

1. High utilization. (The client has already been seen a certain number of times, this number being determined by the benefit plan and type of contract.) Or, requests for a high number or high frequency of sessions.
2. Requesting individual therapy with two members of the same family, or both spouses, at the same time. Or, requesting some combination

of individual, marital, family, and/or group therapy which will lead to higher utilization.

3. Potential denial or uncertainty by the nonclinical assistant/computer algorithm about whether the treatment is still medically necessary.

4. A practitioner whose status has any kind of a "flag" on it due to complaints and/or negative scores on profiling measures. All temporary or ad hoc providers.

5. Incomplete, illegible, and/or un-scannable OTRs.

6. Recent discharge from inpatient, partial hospital, residential, or intensive outpatient treatment.

7. A suspicion of unaddressed substance abuse or medication issues.

8. Personality disorder diagnosis.

9. Complaint by the client or employer.

10. Random audits.

Avoiding as many of these pitfalls as are within your control will help treatment reports sail through without close scrutiny. Probably the most common of these no-no's is leaving blank spaces, or, in an attempt to maintain confidentiality, giving information which is so vague it is worthless. For example, a psychiatrist who sends a treatment report indicating that the client is prescribed "an antidepressant."

Case managers or their assistants are required to call to get information missing from treatment reports. When the assistant or the computer sees a blank space, the OTR gets put in a pile with others that require additional information. This process is laborious and time intensive, frustrating for everyone, and holds up recertification. If the case manager has to call, you've wasted your time, and might as well have scheduled a telephone review. OTRs which pass muster are re-authorized more quickly than those with complications.

If the case manager has to call, you've wasted your time, and might as well have scheduled a telephone review.

> **Survival Tip:** Never send a treatment report which is word-for-word the same as the previous OTR. It will be obvious even if the original date is whited out. If too many sessions have been used or progress isn't evident, the current plan may be compared to the last one submitted. Managed care companies typically retain the paper OTRs, microfilm them, type or scan them into the computer system.

Telephone Review

A few teams in the major companies still make telephone reviews mandatory, but these are more and more of a rarity. It's just too time-consuming, and therefore too expensive. The average OTR can be reviewed and a new certification entered by a case manager in about 15 or 20 minutes, but most telephone reviews take between half an hour and 45 minutes from start to finish, including the case manager's postconversation documentation requirements. Mandatory telephone review is an economic burden on therapists as well. If a therapist has to take an appointment time from his or her schedule for the phone review, that's a loss of income in addition to the reduced per-session rate.

Some managed care account teams allow a choice between a phone review and a written OTR; others completely forbid it, stating they want a request for re-authorization in writing. Or, there may be no specific policy about telephone reviews but the system may disincentivize telephone reviews by making case managers accountable to extremely high turnaround-time or number-completed standards. Therapists who prefer telephone reviews should always call first to verify that this is an available method of obtaining re-authorization.

Therapists who prefer telephone reviews should always call first to verify that this is an available method of obtaining re-authorization.

Survival Tip: Never leave clinical information on the case manager's voice mail to substitute for an OTR or a live telephone review without prior permission from the case manager.

When telephone review is the method of choice, if available:

1. Cases where more than 20–30 sessions have been used and more are still needed (some companies will actually require live reviews anyway after a pre-specified number of sessions).
2. Any case about which there is diagnostic uncertainty.
3. High-risk cases.
4. Medical necessity appears not to be present, but special circumstances in the client's life require continuing treatment. (Be sure not to reveal these without the client's explicit informed consent.)
5. To get to know the case manager. Just don't review an Adjustment Disorder or a very routine case.

6. To request authorization to refer for marital/family therapy, psychiatric evaluation, psychological testing, a higher level of care, group therapy, and so on.

Case Managers as Consultants

Got a clinical question about filling out a written OTR? Consider asking the case manager. He or she is in the best position to know what will or won't be approved. Asking the case manager for advice about how to fill out the treatment report forms is a simple, yet effective way of both building a positive relationship with the managed care company and getting sessions authorized. It conveys an image of *managed care friendliness*.

In telephone reviews, effective case managers ask clinical questions for a reason, and that reason isn't always aimed at denying treatment. When done in a supportive and collegial manner, making a therapist question him- or herself may ultimately be productive for the client—if the therapist is also willing to participate in the process. Of course, there are limits.

Never hesitate to politely ask a case manager in a "live" review why he or she is requesting a particular piece of information.

Never hesitate to politely ask a case manager in a "live" review why he or she is requesting a particular piece of information. There are only two reasons why case managers should be asking questions during the live review:

1. The information they are requesting is necessary to substantiate "medical necessity."
2. The case manager has a hypothesis about the case formulation or treatment plan, and the information is requested to support or disprove the hypothesis. In this event, the therapist has a right to know what the case manager's hypothesis is before answering the question.

"Just curious" is never an acceptable reason for the case manager to request information about a client.

Case managers who are good at their jobs accept that part of it is to take responsibility for setting a collegial and supportive tone to the "live" review.

Case managers who are good at their jobs accept that part of it is to take responsibility for setting a collegial and supportive tone to the "live" review. They understand, or at least acknowledge, therapists' difficulties with managed care.

"Schmoozing" used to be a good strategy (Browning & Browning, 1996). A therapist could get to know the case manager by name, learn something about him or her, and perhaps make a personal connection. While this is all still true in theory, the growth in size and complexity of the managed behavioral care organizations due to the merger frenzy of the middle 1990s has resulted in greater depersonalization of the outpatient utilization review process. Furthermore, the managed care system has set things up such that the case manager is the one with the power, and sometimes case managers have been known to be quite controlling in interaction with therapists. Why?

Far from being treated as respected, experienced professionals, case managers often reveal feeling belittled or even abused in their jobs. Even if one is a therapist, it's a natural human reaction to perceived powerlessness to attempt to find someone weaker to dominate in turn. Former case manager Norman Hering offered this insight when interviewed: "the conflict intrapsychically is that they're looking for . . . power but the company takes it away. Some [case managers] have a desire for power but the position is actually powerless. They are constantly confronted with their powerlessness and [their behavior] is a reaction to this."

Identifying the Abusive Case Manager

It's not always easy to recognize when a problem is the individual case manager, as opposed to managed care in general. No therapist should be subjected to:

- An implication or open statement that no authorization will be given if the therapist disagrees with the case manager.
- Requests for more information than seems necessary.
- Angry, threatening, or defensive behavior if the therapist asks the reason for a request for a particular piece of information, and/or sets boundaries or limits on what will be revealed.
- Someone who doesn't listen well.
- Lectures on how to manage your practice better, write OTRs better, or noncompliance with rules. (It is the job of Provider Relations, not a case manager, to confront panel members about any noncompliance with the company's rules.)
- Orders to take a different approach with a client or change the treatment plan.
- Implications or statements to the effect that "the client would be better by now if you were any good."

- Comments like "if you don't like it, quit!" to a complaint voiced by the therapist.
- Threats to have the therapist removed from the network or officially blackballed. (Be aware that case managers don't typically have the power to carry out these threats.)

"What if I get a case manager who is on a power trip?" Very little can be done during the actual conversation beyond sticking to the main goal of obtaining authorization for the client. Immediately after the review, take a moment to jot down the date, the name of the case manager, and what specifically was objectionable or abusive about his or her conduct. Then, step back a bit and regain some objectivity, because a decision will need to be made as to whether it is worth lodging a formal complaint.

Complaining about a Case Manager's Behavior

Who the therapist should complain to depends on the outcome of the review. If the objectionable behavior occurred during a review that eventually resulted in a denial, the complaint will need to be directed to the Appeals Director. If, however, there was no denial, the therapist will instead be limited to the case manager's supervisor and/or the Clinical Director of the account's case management team. In either case, letters of complaint about case managers should be copied to a vice president or director of Network Management (even if you don't have a name).

If the behavior of the case manager is serious enough to warrant a complaint, it's serious enough that it should be put in writing. Keep the letter simple by giving the name of the case manager, the date of the review, and the name/ID of the client who had been reviewed. (The client's name/ID is important even if there was no denial, because so many reviews occur that it needs to be very clear when and under precisely what circumstances the case manager was inappropriate.) In a factual tone, describe in detail what happened. Then make one of the following requests:

- The case manager be closely telephone monitored to prevent similar behavior from occurring in reviews with other professionals.
- The next time there needs to be a telephone review, to work instead with another case manager or the supervisor. If, for whatever reason, this request absolutely cannot be granted, then request that the next review be silent monitored (live) by the supervisor.
- To send a written OTR instead of doing a telephone review.

Don't request an apology from the case manager. Forced apologies are meaningless and will simply personalize the antagonism.

Alternatives to OTRs

The days are numbered for universal utilization review of outpatient treatment. It's just too expensive; whatever cost savings might be realized by micromanaging outpatient psychotherapy are probably more than eaten up by the administrative costs required. (The managed care companies contacted declined to share figures that would prove or disprove this supposition.) In addition to the fearsome expense of micromanagement is the loss of patients' confidentiality.

The days are numbered for universal utilization review of outpatient treatment.

But what will take the place of OTRs? The issue of outpatient utilization review centers around one critical question: "Does every patient need to be managed and reviewed?" The answer to this question will determine the design of alternative structures. Models in which the answer to the question of reviewing every patient is a "Yes," almost invariably focus on shifting the decision making from the managed care company to the practitioner—with associated financial risk.

The issue of outpatient utilization review centers around one critical question: "Does every patient need to be managed and reviewed?"

Capitation

Inherent in capitation is the ability of the group practice to manage care internally. The advantages are enhanced confidentiality and less interference from the managed care company. But also inherent in any capitated system is a conflict between the economic needs of the practitioner and the treatment needs of the patient (see Chapter 15).

Each capitated group has its own specific UR model. In general, the management of the practice decrees that after a certain specified number of sessions, the clinician will present the case and the treatment plan before a team of his or her peers or the group's UR reviewer, either orally or in writing. Not much different from an OTR or phone review; the only difference is who is making the medical necessity determination.

Provider-Based Utilization Management

There are some experiments underway in returning this function to practicing clinicians, but without the capitated payment structure. Blue Cross/Blue Shield of Minnesota has conceived and implemented a strategy they call "provider-based utilization management" (*Managed Behavioral Health News*, 1998a; *Managed Care Strategies*, 1998b). Groups or community mental health centers (CMHCs) first undergo training to take on the utilization review functions and set up an appeals system.

Blue Cross withholds a certain percentage from the discounted per-session rate, but groups have the opportunity to win it all back. Some of the withheld amounts can be earned back through implementation of quality improvement projects. The rest is put into a pool with the money from the other participating practices. To win it back, each group has to meet a target cost per patient, and its target cost is individualized based on previous performance. The goal is to equalize costs per patient throughout the network. If the group meets the target, it gets the remainder of its own withhold plus a share from practices that did not meet their targets.

Because the numbers are based on groups' previous performance, there is some degree of reality to the financial targets, which is radically different than trying to meet a fixed per-member-per-month rate (PMPM) derived from a competitive bidding process or overtly imposed by the insurer, managed care carve-out company, or HMO. Nor are groups required to take on the enormous infrastructure that frequently accompanies capitation. They are not expected to achieve expensive NCQA accreditation or compliance, because the practice is considered a utilization review "delegate" of the insurer/managed care company, who retains a degree of supervisory control over the groups' UR processes.

Working Smarter, Not Harder: Letting Go of Universal Review

Outcomes-Based Approaches

Recognizing that accountability means results rather than medical necessity, these models do not review every patient. Case managers focus their efforts only on cases where the patient is not progressing, where utilization is higher than average, or on patients with chronic, severe conditions that need careful management to avoid multiple hospitalizations. An additional advantage is that solo practitioners can be used, because the utilization review is still in the hands of the managed care company.

At long last, outcomes are more than just talk. This is where the carveout managed behavioral care companies are putting their efforts. The commonality among the managed care companies' systems is that they all tend to feature outcomes measures taken at various points during treatment, rather than waiting until discharge (Moran, 1998; Managed Care Strategies, 1998a). Instead of a narrative OTR, the therapist completes a checklist. Additionally, there is a questionnaire for the client, made up of self-report measures of symptoms and functioning. It's not totally confidential, but more so than most treatment reports. Like an OTR, the form is required at intervals determined by the company. Although everyone completes the forms, they are computer-scanned and only routed to a case manager if the client is progressing more slowly than what is normative.

Criticisms and Questions

Each company will end up with its own proprietary method; practitioners serving on multiple networks will still have to find ways to keep all the procedures straight. Then there is the question of individual differences and whether or not these systems, such as Compass® (Integra), the OQ-45 (Magellan), the CIMS (MHN-Foundation), or the Life Status Questionnaire (PacifiCare Behavioral), adequately allow for clients who are just plain slower to respond to treatment. How do these systems address the problem of individual circumstances, of which there will always be plenty, without relapsing into universal review? Clients of varying ethnic and cultural backgrounds may differ in the nature and rapidity of their responses, for example. Further study and more in-depth discussion of these questions will have to take place if these real-time outcomes systems are to be depended on for treatment authorization.

Statistical Models

Unlike the outcomes-based measures, the statistical models simply "manage" a predetermined percentage of clients; namely, the most clinically at-risk and the highest utilizers of the system. Atkins (1998) discusses the technique of *statistical process control;* Dubin and O'Brien (1999) describe its implementation with a managed Medicaid population. The selection of patients for focused case management is based on both utilization (the "statistics") and clinical criteria. For example, Dubin and O'Brien report that for the 12 months before beginning the statistical process control model, 30 percent of all inpatient days were used by only 9 percent of all the patients admitted during that year. This means that intensive case management services can be targeted on only 9 percent of covered lives and still affect a third of all inpatient days.

The commonality among the managed care companies' systems is that they all tend to feature outcomes measures taken at various points during treatment, rather than waiting until discharge.

The model is exciting; clinical common sense is reported to correspond well with statistical findings. Naturally, clients with dual-diagnosis, bipolar disorder, schizophrenia, substance abuse, concurrent Axis 2 issues, and severe psychosocial circumstances are going to be at much higher risk and use more costly services than clients with Adjustment Disorder.

A case manager for a managed care company that uses a statistical model, is truly a case manager in the original, pre-managed care sense of the term. He or she follows up to ensure patient compliance, coordinates care provided by professionals of various disciplines and social service agencies, pays attention to the biopsychosocial needs of the patient, and helps him or her to access wrap-around community services. No more gatekeeping, denying, or evaluating the work of colleagues by nit-picking their treatment plans.

9

Completing the Outpatient Treatment Reports

The injunctions to use behaviorally-specific treatment goals and interventions on managed care companies' treatment report forms seem so alien to what we therapists actually do in sessions. Therapy is that experience of being with the client, of instinctually knowing when to keep silent and when to probe, when to confront and when to allow the client the comfort of his or her denial. There is no substitute for the healing power of the therapeutic relationship itself, which cannot be conveyed adequately in a managed care treatment report.

It may help to remember why these reports are being written: to prove the case for medical necessity, so the client can get help paying for treatment. Don't expect that the OTR will reflect the meaning of therapy with the client; it won't.

Don't expect that the OTR will reflect the meaning of therapy with the client; it won't.

Diagnosis

Therapists often ask case managers, "How many sessions does your company give for an Adjustment Disorder?" Or, "Will the client get more sessions if I put down Generalized Anxiety Disorder or Panic Disorder as a diagnosis?" There's a nagging suspicion that the MBHOs have for outpatient psychotherapy what was once known, in the medical field, as DRGs or diagnostic-related groups. Don't ask a case manager this question: If it were really happening, he or she certainly wouldn't be allowed to acknowledge it!

Everyone knows that, for the purposes of insurance reimbursement, not all diagnoses are created equal. There are a few ways to trigger a denial—or an in-depth review of the case—based on diagnosis. V-Codes, for instance, are almost never reimbursed, except in the case of EAP treatment. There are a few plans that will pay for a V-code for the first session, which seems a fair way to ensure diagnostic accuracy, the absence of a permanent mental health record, and the therapist to be paid for his or her work. Over 15 to 20 sessions for any type of Adjustment Disorder is likely to get closer review.

Consistency

The managed care company expects that the diagnosis given on the treatment report be reasonably consistent with the symptoms reported. But there's no need for therapists to be obsessive or paranoid about it. Case managers don't have the time to check to make sure each therapist has listed enough symptoms that meet the criteria for giving the diagnosis. The important point is simply to be sure that the diagnosis chosen fits the symptom profile. It's the very obvious mismatches that will trigger further action:

Be sure that the diagnosis chosen fits the symptom profile.

> Kay Smanager, of HPBH, reviewed an OTR that listed an adult patient's symptoms as irritability, restlessness, anger outbursts, anxiety, ruminating thoughts, and insomnia. But the diagnosis given was Dysthymia. Kay called the therapist to inquire further.

Whatever this patient's diagnosis is, Dysthymia certainly isn't the most obvious choice which comes to mind.

If using a "rule out" or "provisional" diagnosis, there should be at least one definitive diagnosis (even if it's an Adjustment Disorder), that the case manager can enter on the authorization.

> **Survival Tip:** If the diagnosis is really unclear, it's better to qualify it with a "rule out" or "provisional" than it is to be called by a case manager who will ask more probing questions.

If using a "rule out" or "provisional" diagnosis, there should be at least one definitive diagnosis (even if it's an Adjustment Disorder), that the case manager can enter on the authorization. If there are no other diagnoses, a "rule out" may become the "official" diagnosis even though this was not the therapist's intent. Quality Improvement and Clinical Management departments frown on concurrent certifications showing "799.90 Diagnosis Deferred," and will pressure the case manager to use something "real." Therapists also need to use a valid diagnosis for their claim forms, or payment problems will ensue.

Competing Diagnoses

There are some clinical situations in which several diagnoses might be accurate. Choosing one among several plausible diagnoses, in itself, isn't likely to bring about a phone call from the case manager. Instead, case managers will most likely call about issues such as the need for medication or the number of sessions used, and during the conversation, the question of differential diagnosis may well arise.

> GBH case manager Bea Worker called Dina Troy about her OTR for patient Woodrow Alan. Dina had seen Woody 30 times, and was still reporting symptoms of obsessive thoughts, panic attacks, worry, restlessness, agitation, insomnia, fatigue, and difficulty functioning in social situations or in areas with large numbers of people. Woody steadfastly refused to try medication.
>
> Bea questioned whether Dina's diagnosis of Generalized Anxiety Disorder, although certainly matching the symptoms, was the better choice over Social Phobia. She asked many questions about the targeting of Dina's interventions and the source of Woody's anxiety.

This is the sort of situation that rightly leads therapists to conclude that managed care is interfering in treatment decisions. Just a cursory look at the *DSM-IV* would reveal that a diagnosis of Generalized Anxiety disorder is a highly appropriate choice. The only differentiating factor between this and Social Phobia would be whether or not other things besides social situations trigger Woody's anxiety, and this information isn't always going to be readily available from a treatment report.

There's really no way Dina could have avoided the case manager's call; Bea was just doing her job. GBH might have a policy that case managers conduct more intensive reviews after a certain number of sessions—or if the patient refuses medication. All any therapist can do when questioned by a case manager is to simply articulate the reasons why one diagnosis was chosen over other plausible alternatives. And don't worry; additional treatment should *never* be denied on the grounds of differential diagnosis.

Additional treatment should never be denied on the grounds of differential diagnosis.

Common Diagnostic Pitfalls

Axis I: Include the Modifiers

When diagnosing Major Depression or Bipolar Disorder, the specific number code indicates diagnostic differences among subtypes of these disorders. These *modifiers*, found after the decimal point, and which no one can ever remember without flipping through the *DSM-IV*, mean something that the case manager is going to want. For Depression, the first digit differentiates between single episode and recurrent; for Bipolar Disorders, those numbers characterize the "manic" or "depressive" nature of the most recent episode. The second digit, in both cases, is a severity index.

Isn't this kind of trivial? Clinically, maybe. It's certainly not always easy to determine which "bipolar disorder" diagnosis is the most accurate, and the distinction isn't that useful when doing therapy. Procedurally, though, a complete diagnosis must be entered into the managed care company's computer in order to issue authorizations and to pay claims. The case manager or assistant entering the data has only two options if a therapist leaves off a modifier. One is to call the therapist for clarification; the other is to guess. Remember the numbers involved on the managed care company's end. Chances are good that, no matter how unethical or wrong it might be to guess, the managed care employee will do it because s/he is just too overwhelmed to call every single practitioner who leaves a modifier off a diagnosis code. Avoid having an erroneous diagnosis entered into the client's permanent medical record by making sure to include modifier codes where specified by the *DSM-IV*.

Avoid having an erroneous diagnosis entered into the client's permanent medical record by making sure to include modifier codes where specified by the DSM-IV.

"Polysubstance Abuse" is not a *DSM-IV* diagnosis. If the client doesn't meet the criteria for Polysubstance Dependence, choose instead the one or two most favored drugs and diagnose as Alcohol Abuse, Cocaine Abuse, and so on, assuming the client meets *DSM-IV* criteria. It's always possible to specify in a side comment what other drugs are being used.

Case managers reviewing outpatient treatment reports not only frequently see the notation of "alcoholism," but also "alcohol" or "marijuana," with no clarification. Alcohol what? Social use only? *DSM-IV* requires the clinician to specify: abuse, dependence, intoxication, delirium, or withdrawal. Therapists who identify a substance without clarification tend to look passive-aggressive and managed-care unfriendly.

Why should case managers want to refer clients to someone who makes their job harder?

Is it wrong to list more than two Axis I diagnoses on an OTR? Not from the standpoint of the case manager reviewing the OTR. It's wise, though, not to list diagnoses that aren't actively being treated. A diagnosis appearing on the OTR but not among the treatment goals is likely to trigger a call from the case manager, who will want to know why. This is especially true if the diagnosis concerns substance abuse (see Chapter 11).

It's wise not to list diagnoses that aren't actively being treated.

> Kay Smanager reviewed a treatment plan for Joe Schmoe. Dina Troy had listed a diagnosis of Major Depression Recurrent Moderate, and Alcohol Dependence, Full Remission. Joe's goals were: (1) to improve mood, sleep, appetite; and (2) to improve marital/family communication. Dina did not give any specifics about Joe's drinking/treatment history, the length of his sobriety, or the nature of his involvement with AA.
>
> Kay was obligated to call to get the above information. HPBH had promised Joe's employer that 99 percent of all clients with substance abuse diagnoses would receive referral to 12-step groups.

What if Joe Schmoe had been sober for 10 years? Is it ethically appropriate for Dina to have perpetuated the alcohol diagnosis on his medical record, given that the problems for which Joe was seeking help now were not directly related to his past history of drinking or present-day relapse prevention?

More is definitely NOT always better. In terms of confidentiality, listing a diagnosis that isn't part of the treatment plan is revealing some aspect of the client's life that is irrelevant to the determination of "medical necessity" for the current episode of therapy.

More is definitely not always better.

Axis II

Diagnosing a personality disorder on Axis II should be the exception, rather than the rule (see Chapter 11).

Axis III

Many therapists ignore this section, but a complete OTR makes for a happy case manager and faster re-authorization. If the client is healthy, write "none," "healthy," or "no medical problems," in this field. It may

Given NCQA's mandate of coordination with primary care look for an increasing emphasis on completion of Axis III.

seem trivial, but given NCQA's mandate of coordination with primary care (NCQA, 1998, QI 6.2; 2000, QI 8), look for an increasing emphasis on completion of Axis III.

Other therapists tend to use Axis III to list symptoms of the Axis I disorder.

> Axis I. 296.23 Major Depression, Single Episode, Severe
> Axis II. 799.90 Deferred
> Axis III. interrupted sleep, weight gain
> Axis IV. problems with primary support
> Axis V. Current 45; past year 70

Axis III is used for General Medical Conditions (APA, 1994). All OTR forms have a checklist or place to identify the symptoms supporting the Axis I diagnosis. Listing symptoms contributing to Axis I on Axis III might be misinterpreted as a medical problem, which could have negative consequences for authorization. Interrupted sleep, for example, is a symptom of Major Depression, but there are medical conditions, such as sleep apnea, which also cause interruptions in sleep. It certainly doesn't do any good if the case manager concludes that the client needs medical treatment instead of psychotherapy.

Axis IV

Case managers appreciate it when therapists specify the client's stressors on Axis IV even further than what the current DSM-IV categories allow.

"Mild," "moderate," and "severe" descriptors of psychosocial stressors were last seen in the *DSM-III-R*. Use the *DSM-IV* system of characterizing stressors according to their nature, not the *DSM-III-R* method of characterizing them according to severity. Or, do both. Case managers appreciate it when therapists specify the client's stressors on Axis IV even further than what the current *DSM-IV* categories allow. "Problems with primary support" can be narrowed to "marital conflict," or "economic problems" can be specified as "bankruptcy" or "nonpayment of child support."

Axis V

Probably at least two-thirds of therapists don't list Axis V ratings when they submit OTRs. It's uncomfortable to know that what is a subjective assessment of the client's functioning is going to become part of the "official" diagnosis. There are also many of us who never use the GAF except for purposes of managed care, because the system isn't very meaningful to the actual process of psychotherapy. But if a GAF must be entered into the managed care company computer, better it be what the therapist assesses than a guess by the case manager or a non-clinical assistant or data entry clerk. Because managed care employees don't have the time to call 60 percent of the therapists submitting OTRs to ask what is the GAF, guessing is rampant.

Why can't they just put "0" and be done with it! Many times that's exactly what the managed care employees do. After all, "0" is what the APA (1994) has designated as the GAF score when there is not sufficient information to make an assessment of global functioning. But that only works until QI initiatives occur and case managers are pestered with reminders to include a "real" GAF. Even if the therapist puts "0" (as opposed to leaving a blank space), case managers might be forced to guess—or call each and every therapist.

GAF scores are generally expected to be no higher than the mild symptoms range (61 through 70) for outpatient clients whose treatment is medically necessary.

Are they going to deny if the GAF Score is too high? Although I've never known of any instance where the GAF score was the reason for either certification or denial of outpatient treatment, it is sometimes mentioned as a factor in companies' medical necessity guidelines. GAF scores are generally expected to be no higher than the mild symptoms range (61 through 70) for outpatient clients whose treatment is medically necessary.

Clinical Presentation/Psychosocial History Section

Thankfully, not every OTR requires a narrative summary. But when there is a form that does, do you stare at the blank space, wondering what to write that will get the patient authorization, but without revealing too much?

Focus on current symptoms and problems functioning. This is the managed care company "formula" for medical necessity (see Chapter 7). Start by answering the question, "What symptoms is the client displaying which supports the choice of diagnosis?" Next, identify the life areas in which the symptoms are causing difficulty, and (briefly) outline the nature of the difficulty. Only reveal whatever extraneous details are absolutely necessary to understand the client's presenting problem. Then, mention whatever stressors or life circumstances are contributing to the issue(s). If the symptom profile seems weak, describe the problems for which the patient is seeking treatment and what is known to be causing the difficulties.

In summary:

- *Be brief.* "Just the facts, ma'am," as that old TV detective used to say.
- *Stick to the facts.* Hypotheses about "why" the client feels the way he or she does aren't facts, and they aren't what managed care considers medically necessary. Concentrate on "what" is observably wrong.
- *Don't second-guess the form.* It says what it says. What it doesn't ask for, don't answer.
- *Assume that every word written in the Clinical Synopsis paragraph will be typed or scanned word for word into the managed care company's computer.*

According to these principles, why is summary A clearly more effective than summary B for the purposes of managed care reauthorization?

Please give a short clinical formulation. Explain symptoms, stressors, factors related to treatment, psychosocial issues, functioning, and relevant patient history. Why is continued treatment medically necessary?

A. Cindy is tearful, reports irritability, fatigue, insomnia, hopelessness, and depressed mood. Denies suicidal ideation and/or plan and has no history of same. Panic attacks two or three times a week w/high continuous level of anxiety. Nightmares at times. Worries, reports racing thoughts which interfere with concentration on the job. Reports less patience with parenting her 10-year-old son. Difficulty saying no to others which results in feelings of resentment and being overwhelmed. Angry at husband's emotional distance and unable to let him know what she needs. No alcohol, illicit drug, or prescription drug use.

B. Cindy is depressed, angry, has low self-esteem, and compensates for lack of attention from husband with workaholic behavior. Tends to get herself trapped in interpersonal dynamics in which she is repeatedly taken advantage of/victimized. Panic attacks, depression, anxiety all stem from repression of past abuse. No history of suicide attempts and isn't suicidal now. Reports nightmares but is resistant to discussing their content. Poor insight into her problems and those of her family. Problems with work and parenting. No substance abuse.

More symptoms are mentioned in summary A. Summary B hypothesizes that the origin of the symptoms is childhood abuse. It also implies that treatment of the symptoms should be a "corrective emotional experience" of uncovering all the painful baggage of childhood abuse—not an approach managed care would favor.

Playing the Game

Am I saying that therapists should change their way of practicing to please managed care? No. It's better advocacy for a client, though, not to advertise any treatment or philosophical orientation that will force a confrontation with the biases of the payor. It may well be that the managed care company will deny the client's sessions before treatment is concluded; but there's no reason for the therapist to hasten that denial.

It's better advocacy for a client not to advertise any treatment or philosophical orientation that will force a confrontation with the biases of the payor.

The symptoms in A are more specific. "Depressed" is operationalized into "tearful, irritability, fatigue, insomnia, hopelessness, and depressed mood." Likewise, in A the panic attacks are specified as having a frequency of 2 or 3 times per week; there is no frequency given in B. Although frequency isn't a requirement of "medical necessity" *per se*, identifying the current frequency or intensity of symptoms makes it a lot easier to write the treatment goals (see Chapter 10).

In terms of functioning, A is again more specific. Instead of saying "problems with work and parenting," A outlines that the client has difficulty concentrating and decreased patience and ties these symptoms to decreased functioning in the relevant life areas.

Once again, more is not always better. It's also instructive to note that the more effective summary, A, actually reveals *less* information about the client. Summary B indicates she's a survivor of childhood abuse; summary A does not.

Stay Present-Focused

There are only two circumstances in which the family background issues of an adult client should be revealed in a managed care treatment plan:

1. The family issues *directly* impact on the client's present impairment in functioning.

2. To establish genetic loading for diagnoses (especially important for obtaining benefits for clients with "biologically-based" disorders under mental health parity laws).

But our past is who we are, says innate therapist wisdom, so diametrically opposed to this cut-and-dried managed care approach. How can the distinction be made as to whether the past event(s) *directly* impacts current functioning? Use a very common-sense, writer's guideline: If the case manager would not understand the presentation without revealing the past event, then include that past event or circumstance. Otherwise, don't.

"Saying a client has low self-esteem is the kiss of death," says former case manager Norman Hering.

Avoid traditional psychotherapy terms. "Saying a client has low self-esteem is the kiss of death," says former case manager Norman Hering, who went on to add, "Managed care companies don't see low self-esteem as 'medically necessary.'" Terms that connote "quality of life" therapy, long-term therapy, or psychoanalysis should be avoided at all cost when completing a managed care treatment report.

The Psychotherapy-to-Managed Care Dictionary

Table 9.1, wherever possible, suggests alternative language or phrasing that can be used on treatment reports in place of traditional terms. Why is using managed care lingo so important? It's the "pass muster" phenomenon: on the surface, reports which look "managed care-compliant" are less likely to be questioned, and more likely to be quickly approved (see Chapter 8).

On the surface, reports which look "managed care-compliant" are less likely to be questioned, and more likely to be quickly approved.

(User's note: The "translations" will seem inadequate, because many of these concepts don't exist in the "Managed Care" worldview. This dictionary is solely for use as an aid to completing OTR's and in telephone reviews to get sessions for clients using managed care benefits.)

Practicalities

When reading the answers to free-form questions on treatment reports, case managers don't take points off for incomplete sentences, bad grammar, or incorrect spelling. There is very little space for answers, so it's best to use only words that are absolutely necessary. But the managed

Table 9.1
Psychotherapy to Managed Care Dictionary

Traditional Psychotherapy terms:	Managed care "translations:"
Analysis; analyze (verb; intervention)	Educate; explore options; help client identify; help client verbalize.
Catharsis (concept/theoretical construct)	(Note: there is no translation of the actual concept in the managed care world-view. However, there is a rough translation in a form which can be used as an intervention.) [Allow/encourage/teach/help] patient to [vent/express/identify/release/verbalize] feelings.
Client-centered therapy (intervention; therapeutic orientation)	Intervention: Provide safe place for client to express and identify feelings; encourage client to identify/express feelings; reflect client's expressions of feelings in nonjudgmental manner.
Corrective emotional experience (intervention)	(This is "iffy" to use, even in the "translation," because the whole idea of a "corrective emotional experience" still depends on the therapeutic relationship and/or experience of being in therapy, neither of which is valued much in the managed care paradigm.) Intervention: Client will learn about healthy relationships through [therapeutic relationship; demonstrations of warmth; caring; openness; honesty; genuineness; unconditional positive regard].
Dream work (intervention)	No known translation. (If you're doing this, don't mention it on the OTR!)
Dynamics (concept/theoretical construct)	(Spell out the nature of the interpersonal relationships or the intrapersonal issues, avoiding the word "dynamics," which connotes longterm, insight-oriented therapy or psychoanalysis). For example: Client and spouse tend to relate in an approach-avoid, pursuer-distancer pattern. Or: Client tends to bury his anger and resentment at his boss until he gets home, then lets it out at his wife and family.
Dysfunctional family (concept/theoretical construct)	[Alcoholic/chemically dependent] family; [physically/sexually/verbally/emotionally abusive family]; emotionally distant family; family exhibits lack of interpersonal boundaries; divorced parents are hostile toward each other and place the children in the middle; father abandoned mother; client does not know biological mother; etc.
Ego (concept/theoretical construct)	Instead, consider using one of the following, depending on how you're using the word "ego": self; impulse control (for the ego function of mediating between id and superego); identity; consciousness; conscious awareness.

(continued)

Table 9.1 (Continued)

Traditional Psychotherapy terms:	Managed care "translations:"
Enmeshed (clinical description; adjective)	Clinical Description: Weak boundaries [between spouses; in family] as evidenced by [spouses will answer for the other; no knocking on doors; parents look through children's diaries; when a family member/spouse feels a certain way the expectation is that the other spouse/family members will feel the same]. Goal: [relate to specific problem identified above] Parents to report no more reading children's diaries; each spouse to demonstrate speaking only for him/herself in marital therapy, etc. Intervention: In family/marital therapy, [educate; reflect; confront; identify] [specific problems as reported under Clinical Description]. Intervention: In family/marital therapy, [teach; demonstrate; role-play; develop] alternative ways of relating; [then specify according to problem identified earlier, i.e., each spouse to speak for self; establish privacy norms in family, etc.]
Id (concept/theoretical construct)	Clinical Description (overfunctioning): Patient behaves according to impulses without thinking through the potential consequences. Becomes angry if not allowed to satisfy impulses. Clinical Description (underfunctioning): Patient does not allow him- or herself to have fun, relax, be child-like or spontaneous.
Insight; develop insight (concept/theoretical construct; intervention)	Clinical Description: Client [is unable; has trouble; struggles] to [articulate, verbalize; express; understand; identify; state] [insert the issue/problem client has no insight about]. Goal: [Instead of using combinations of the above words to equal "develop insight," the goal should focus on the problem itself. I.e., your goal will state "client will eliminate physically aggressive behavior" rather than "client will develop insight into his physically aggressive behavior."] Intervention: Help client [identify; articulate; understand; verbalize; express; state] [triggers of problem/behavior; factors influencing problem/behavior; alternative approaches to problem/behavior]. (Warning: Make sure this is listed as one of several interventions for the same goal . . . managed care does not like to pay for "developing insight.")
Intellectualization (clinical description; defense mechanism)	Clinical Description: Patient avoids expression of feelings by discussing thoughts or rational, demonstrable phenomena. Goal: Patient to express feelings using feeling words such as [angry, sad, scared, lonely, joyous, irritated, bewildered]. Intervention: [teach; demonstrate; identify; practice] range and vocabulary of feelings; [identify; pinpoint; address; confront] obstacles to expressing feelings. [Practice; role-play; encourage; facilitate] expressions of feelings.
Narcissism; Narcissistic (clinical description; adjective)	Clinical Description: Client tends to be preoccupied with him/herself; seems to lack empathy for others; is often grandiose; wants continuous admiration; high sense of his/her own importance; expects others to comply with his/her every wish.

Table 9.1 (Continued)

Traditional Psychotherapy terms:	Managed care "translations:"
Overcome denial (Goal; intervention)	*Intervention:* [confront; examine] denial regarding [substance abuse, violent behavior, passive-aggressive behavior, effects of physical abuse by husband, etc.]. *Intervention:* Educate regarding [substance abuse, violent behavior, passive-aggressive behavior, effects of domestic violence, etc.]. *Goal:* Patient will verbalize [understanding, awareness] of [dangerousness, damaging, self-harmful] nature of [problem]. *Goal:* patient will [express, state, verbalize, report, develop] motivation to change as evidenced by action plan to [patient's action which will bring about change].
Projection (defense mechanism)	*Clinical Description:* Client [seems; tends] to [attribute; ascribe; perceive; interpret] others' [opinions, feelings; attitudes, behaviors] in light of her own [opinions, feelings; attitudes, behaviors]. *Intervention:* Teach client to [identify; verbalize; recognize] his/her own [opinions, feelings; attitudes, behaviors]. *Intervention:* [Practice; teach; role-play] cognitive reframing of perceptions in interpersonal relationships.
Rationalize; Rationalization (verb; defense mechanism)	*Clinical Description:* Patient seems unable to accept his/her actions without finding intellectual, interpersonal, or external "reasons" to support these actions. *Intervention:* Teach client to [identify; verbalize; recognize] his/her own [opinions, feelings; attitudes, behaviors] and accept their validity through cognitive restructuring techniques such as [list].
Re-parenting (intervention or therapeutic technique)	*(Note: Even in its managed care form, this still strongly implies long-term therapy to most case managers!)* *Goal:* patient to learn through therapeutic relationship that relationships do not have to be [abusive; critical; controlling]. *Intervention:* [Convey; provide; demonstrate to patient] [Support; encourage; nonjudgmental; approval; kindness; compassion; warmth; caring; concern].
Repression; Repressed (verb; defense mechanism adjective)	Client does not acknowledge [fact, event, etc.]; Patient seems unaware of [face, event, etc.]; Client does not verbalize [fact, event, etc.]; Patient may not be able to access memories of [fact, event, etc.];
Resistance; Going with the resistance (concept/theoretical construct; intervention)	*Client Description:* Patient [and/or couple, family] [show ambivalence; are hesitant; find excuses not to make progress; block themselves; continuously offer reasons to the contrary]. *Intervention:* Help patient [and/or couple, family] achieve goals through ["Prescribing the symptom"; exploring why change is a bad idea; identifying negative aspects of change; other paradoxical techniques].

(continued)

Table 9.1 (Continued)

Traditional Psychotherapy terms:	Managed care "translations:"
Resolve unfinished issues [with one's parents, surrounding a significant event, etc.] (Clinical description; Goal; Intervention)	*Clinical Description:* Patient indicates that [event/issue] continues to have negative impact on current functioning, due to [specify symptoms]. *Goal:* Patient to [report, verbalize, demonstrate, indicate] resolution of [event/issue], as evidenced by [symptoms; no more than 1 nightmare per week, improved mood 5 out of 7 days per week, a reduction of 10 points on the BDI, etc.]. *Goal:* Patient to verbalize awareness that she has control over current mood and anxiety level; patient to identify that she does not have to let [memories of event/issue] influence current mood or functioning; patient to report being able to stop intrusion/flooding of memories at will. *Intervention:* [Teach; educate; identify] [what triggers bring back memories of event; how patient keeps trauma alive; how patient has blocked her ability to let go; practice relaxation; practice meditation; practice letting go; other exercises to disconnect past and present].
Self-Esteem (concept/theoretical construct) Improve/Develop/Raise Self-Esteem (Goal/intervention)	*Clinical Description:* Patient tends to make frequent statements about his/her [inadequacies, failures, inability to achieve positive results, self-blame, refers to other people being "better," accepts responsibility for things that go wrong but not for things that go right.] *Goal:* Patient to [report, demonstrate, display, evidence, make] fewer [negative self-statements, expressions of "I can't," expressions of self-blame, personalizing statements, all-or-nothing statements, expressions of personal failure]. *Intervention:* [Teach; practice; role-play; demonstrate] [errors of attribution, talking back to irrational thoughts, reframing, breaking down lofty goals into achievable parts, how patient's self-talk becomes a self-fulfilling prophecy, daily affirmations].
Superego (concept/theoretical construct)	*Clinical Description* (overfunctioning): Patient unable to relax or allow self to have fun; is rigid and highly concerned with rules and protocol; has difficulty identifying humor in situations. *Clinical Description* (underfunctioning): Patient tends to ignore the rights of others, rules of society, others' feelings and needs in order to fulfill own wishes and desires.
Therapeutic relationship; Therapeutic alliance (concept/theoretical construct; intervention)	*Concept:* There is no known translation. *Intervention:* Listening, empathy, providing support, encouraging client to express feelings, expressions of concern.
Transference; countertransference (concept/theoretical construct; intervention)	No known translation acceptable for use on a managed care treatment report.
Unconscious (concept/theoretical construct)	[Educate about; reflect; confront; identify; pinpoint] patterns of [thinking; behavior; interpersonal interaction] which contribute to the presenting issue.

care employees (or computers) do need to be able to read it, so legibility is key.

Second and Subsequent Treatment Reports

Include a brief description of the client's progress and what remains to be achieved before the client is ready for discharge. Note prominently any relapses or obstacles to achieving the goals, but without theorizing why. Just state what progress has or hasn't been made, or what obstacles have gotten in the way, and what progress must be achieved before the client can safely be discharged from therapy.

Depending on the form, "progress" may be requested in the goals and interventions section, or it may be requested as part of a free-form clinical synopsis. Often there is a Likert-type rating scale rather than a narrative description. Either way, the trick is to indicate enough progress such that therapy is perceived to have benefit, but not so much that the managed care company concludes that the client is ready to be discharged (see Chapter 10).

The trick is to indicate enough progress such that therapy is perceived to have benefit, but not so much that the managed care company concludes that the client is ready to be discharged.

Introduce a new problem. If applicable, describing new problems is vital, even if the "new" problem is highly related to the original problem. The important point is that the justification for the additional sessions should be concrete, and be phrased using the symptoms and impaired functioning mantra that the codes of medical necessity are most likely to understand and accept.

A clinical presentation summary for a second or subsequent OTR that introduces a new problem and discusses progress, might look like this:

> Cindy remains anxious and reports panic attacks about once weekly, although the symptoms of depression, tearfulness, irritability, fatigue, and hopelessness have improved since she was prescribed Paxil. Initial and middle insomnia continues to be a problem and is being addressed with her psychiatrist. Is beginning to report improved communication with her husband about her needs and feelings, but remains highly anxious and fearful of his rejection. New problem is her conflict with her new supervisor at work. Cindy feels belittled and intimidated by this woman who she describes as critical and impatient, and who has unrealistic expectations for the amount of work client can handle. Client is afraid to bring her concerns to her boss and is frantically looking for a new job.

Don't Ever Reveal to the Managed Care Company . . .

The client may have signed the intake form which says "I authorize Dr. Therapist to release whatever information about me is necessary to obtain insurance reimbursement," but practitioners can't be too careful about disclosing these issues to a case manager in a telephone conversation or on a written treatment report:

- Deviant sexual behavior (paraphilias, etc.).
- HIV status.
- Homosexuality.
- Gender identity disorder.
- Criminal behavior for which the client was not caught.
- Criminal convictions not relevant to diagnosis, presenting problems, or treatment plan.
- Other stigmatizing medical conditions such as sexually transmitted diseases.
- Unsubstantiated allegations of child abuse.
- Allegations concerning the behavior of an ex or separated spouse, particularly when children are involved.
- Past victim of sexual abuse, rape, or other sexual trauma.
- Extramarital affairs.
- Sexual harassment (victim or perpetrator) in a work situation.
- Financial information (amount of salary, amount of debt, amount of child support, etc.).

But what if medical necessity can't be demonstrated without releasing something potentially dangerous?

But what if medical necessity can't be demonstrated without releasing something potentially dangerous? Occasionally, it does happen. Clients may be relatively asymptomatic and functioning reasonably well, but if the central issue of therapy is, say, the client's concerns about sexual preference, an extramarital affair, or past sexual trauma, it's going to be pretty hard to substantiate "medical necessity" without revealing the central issue. What does a therapist do then?

Justa Therapist sees Cliff Carson for the first time. Cliff presented with anxiety due to discovering he is infected with genital herpes. Ashamed, he admitted having an affair with a woman at his job, one of his subordinates, and that the affair was still going on. Worse, said Cliff, he has had sex with his wife since sleeping with the woman from work, and now is terrified that his wife will get herpes as well and know that he's been unfaithful. Other than Cliff's anxiety, which seemed in proportion to the situation, there were no significant symptoms.

Dr. Therapist was allowed two sessions with Cliff by his managed behavioral care organization, HPBH, and a treatment report was required to obtain additional sessions beyond that point.

Dr. Therapist is in a bind if Cliff wants more than the two sessions authorized by HPBH. If she doesn't reveal the information, there might be a denial. Revealing the information, though, risks serious negative consequences for Cliff. It's likely that Cliff would be smart and realize that his best bet is to pay Dr. Therapist cash, but what if he were to insist on using his insurance?

Delay the inevitable "point of no return" as long as possible. Dr. Therapist should start by sending in a treatment plan that does not reveal the information. Possibly a few more sessions might be squeezed out of them. In the Clinical Synopsis section of the OTR, she might write,

Delay the inevitable "point of no return" as long as possible.

> 45-year-old married male, anxious about marital problems. Work performance, specifically interpersonal interactions with female subordinates, has been impaired.

Even though Cliff's performance of his job tasks might not have been affected, a supervisor and a subordinate having a sexual liaison can be certainly be called an interpersonal impairment—of extreme degree.

Would the managed care company authorize more sessions based on this one rather vague sentence? Of course, that's going to depend on factors such as the benefit plan and the type of contract Cliff's employer and HPBH have signed (see Chapter 7), but if only two sessions have been authorized it's likely that Cliff would get at least two or three more. Better than nothing, at any rate. What this does is buy Dr. Therapist more time to build the therapeutic alliance and educate Cliff about the threats to his privacy inherent in using his insurance. If necessary, she should show him the treatment plan that reveals the "hot" information (and document having done so) before actually sending it, to give him one last chance to give or withhold consent.

Risk

If the therapist can show to the managed care company that the client is at risk to himself or herself and/or others in any way, re-authorization is assured.

Every OTR has a risk section, even if it's just a checklist. In many ways, risk is what it's all about. If the therapist can show to the managed care company that the client is at risk to himself or herself and/or others in any way, re-authorization is assured. However, the majority of outpatient therapy clients aren't actively suicidal or homicidal. If they are, they usually don't stay outpatient for very long. There are, though, several varieties of risk factor in addition to "suicidal/homicidal" or the more generic "dangerous to self/others." Other risk areas to consider:

- *Any history of suicide attempt.* It doesn't matter how long ago it was. If the detail is available, describe how the attempt was made and what triggered it. Even if the patient is denying suicidal ideation or plan at the moment, suicide attempt in the past is a serious risk indicator and it increases the perception of risk in the case manager's mind.

- *Any family history of completed or attempted suicide.* If someone in the client's family suicided, or made attempts, it's commonly accepted that this places a client at higher risk.

- *Current suicidal ideation without plan.* Note it even if there's low likelihood that the patient will act on his/her thoughts. It's not lying, if the patient has reported thoughts of suicide and/or death.

- *Past history of aggressive or violent behavior.* Past violence is a good predictor of future violence. It's almost a guarantee of getting needed authorization.

- *Present aggressive or violent behavior.* The classic dangerous to others, even if not overtly homicidal.

- *Poor impulse control.* Impulse control is crucial in determining risk. It's like a wild card—if the patient is impulsive, how can professionals predict dangerousness with any degree of certainty? Lack of impulse control is what may cause one patient to attempt and complete suicide while another refrains. Furthermore, even a reasonable degree of impulse control can be lessened through the use of alcohol and drugs.

- *Child abuse.* Be careful. Unless the therapist specifies that what is being commented on in the OTR is not legally reportable, the case manager will be on the phone to the therapist in a flash. Case managers, too, are mandatory reporters. If the abuse is reportable, don't mention it on an OTR unless the report has already been made—don't get managed care involved in the needing to make a report.

Managed care typically considers that family situations with verbal and emotional abuse, although not reportable, are at least mild risk situations. It's also okay to state on a treatment report that something is suspected but not known for sure—as long as the suspicion is clearly labeled as such. If mentioning suspicions, state what is causing you to have these suspicions.

If the abuse is reportable, don't mention it on an OTR unless the report has already been made— don't get managed care involved in the needing to make a report.

- *Elder abuse.* Same as with child abuse. Although not every state may have a law concerning mandatory reporting of elder abuse, it is a risk to another individual.

- *Domestic violence.* Domestic violence can be defined more broadly than just the classic "battered woman" scenario. Consider domestic violence as any physical aggressiveness or property damage perpetrated by one capable adult of either gender, against another capable adult of either gender. As with child abuse, if you suspect "something is going on," it's okay to report those suspicions, as long as they are labeled as such.

- *Risks due to chemical dependency.* Alcoholic clients who are known to the therapist to drink and drive are a risk to themselves and others. Drug-using clients are always at risk for legal charges of possession and distribution. Using on the job risks loss of job and, in some occupations, poses a safety risk to self and others.

- *Medical complications.* This can be any of a number of issues, and is perhaps the most overlooked of the risk factors. A thorough assessment might reveal any number of medical complications that can be used to support the case for "medical necessity." For example, stress-related conditions such as hypertension, cardiac problems, asthma, diabetes, irritable bowel syndrome, and fibromyalgia should be mentioned, along with the potential medical risks to the patient if mental health treatment is discontinued. Other medical conditions that might be a factor for concern are any in which lifestyle and emotional issues can help or hinder medical treatment. Obesity is a common example.

- Eating disorders such as anorexia and bulimia, and the potential accompanying medical complications (i.e., malnutrition, amenorrhea, electrolyte imbalances, dental decay, abuse of laxatives or diuretics), are risk factors.

Not about to Risk Malpractice over Some Job

Just like any other clinician, the last thing a case manager wants is to get sued for malpractice.

Like private practitioners, case managers have to maintain licensure and malpractice insurance. Many of them have part-time private practices. Just like any other clinician, the last thing a case manager wants is to get sued for malpractice. This can be used to the client's advantage, and will become even more of a factor as patients are increasingly being granted the legal right to sue managed care companies.

Be sure to include a safety plan wherever risk is reported. Many therapists assume that the case manager knows what they're going to do. Which is a reasonable assumption, but not all OTRs are reviewed by clinicians (see Chapter 8). Furthermore, the managed care company, ever sensitive to its own liability, still expects the therapist to be the one to spell it all out. Reporting risk may increase the chances of getting authorization, but not reporting a safety plan increases the chances of getting a phone call from the case manager.

Safety plans are so automatic, therapists forget that they are actually interventions that demonstrate accountability (see Table 9.2). How many therapists give a second thought to having a pager and telling a client to call if feeling suicidal? Yet that is a safety plan, and should be documented. "If it isn't documented, it didn't happen," is the motto of managed care.

When in doubt, assume risk to be present and worth mentioning

Not sure if something should be considered a risk factor? When in doubt, assume risk to be present and worth mentioning.

Symptom Checklists and Rating Scales

Preformatted symptom profiles come in two types: the checklist and the Likert-type rating scale. Both are quick and easy for computers to score, and are increasingly used as part of the recertification process.

Table 9.2
Common Interventions for Risk Situations

Risk Factor	Safety Plan/Intervention
Suicide/Risk to self	• Pt contracted to page this therapist 24 × 7 if thinking about ways to commit suicide.
	• Pt contracted to go to the emergency room if having suicidal thoughts or plan.
	• Pt agreed to allow spouse to remove weapons from the house and put them in hiding.
	• Pt agreed to call a suicide hotline if having thoughts of wanting to die.
	• Pt was given the number of a suicide hotline.
	• Pt agreed to allow spouse to administer medication.
	• Pt agreed to go to the emergency room if feeling the impulse to cut on self/burn self or self-mutilate in other ways.
Homicide/Risk to others	• Pt contracted to call a cab [the police, 911] to get to the emergency room if having thoughts of hurting or killing others.
	• Pt agreed to page this therapist 24 × 7 if having thoughts or a plan of hurting or killing others.
	• Pt agreed to allow spouse to remove all weapons from the home.
Poor impulse control	• Pt made list of situations likely to result in [impulsive behavior; i.e., gambling, violence, overspending, substance abuse, reckless driving, etc.]
	• Pt agreed to go to a 12-step meeting [contact sponsor] if in a situation likely to result in the addictive or impulsive behavior.
	• Pt contracted to call a friend [exercise, go to a movie, etc.] if stressed and about to engage in impulsive behavior.
	• Pt to practice relaxation exercises at the three most stressful times of the day.
Child/Elder abuse	• Explored alternative placement options for [mother/father] such as assisted living or skilled nursing facilities.
	• Agreed to allow spouse to handle child/eldercare when feeling anger build.
	• Pt contracted to leave house and go for a walk or work out when feeling anger explosion imminent.
	• Pt given information regarding community respite/crisis nursery programs.
	• Pt referred to Parents Anonymous.
	• Pt given number of hotline(s) to call when angry.

(continued)

Table 9.2 (Continued)

Risk Factor	Safety Plan/Intervention
Domestic violence	• Pt was given the numbers of local hotlines and encouraged to call as needed. • Pt was instructed to keep change of clothing and important papers in trunk of her car in case she needs to leave in a hurry. • Advised pt of her right to call the police if husband becomes violent. • Explained how to obtain an order of protection. • Gave information about shelters if needing a place to stay. • Helped pt identify where she can go if needing to leave. • Pt agreed to leave house [work out, take 10 deep breaths, etc.] if about to explode.
Substance abuse	• Pt agreed to allow spouse to take keys when drinking. • Pt agreed to call sponsor/go to meeting if unable to refrain from drinking/using. • Went over written relapse prevention plan and helped pt structure time with healthy activities such as [list] • Confronted regarding potential consequences of continued use.
Medical complications	• Pt agreed to check blood pressure/blood sugars/heart rate etc. X times per day as recommended by MD. • Pt has been referred to a nutritionist to develop meal plan. • Pt contracted to exercise for at least 20 minutes per day, 3 days/week, [or other time period] by [nature of exercise]. • Pt has been educated regarding the need for medication compliance. • Pt will talk to MD about side effects of [name of medication]. • Pt will keep next appointment with MD. • Pt encouraged to consult with MD before stopping medications. • Pt has been referred to his or her primary care physician to rule out cardiac problems [for panic attacks]. • Pt agrees to carry asthma inhaler at all times. • Pt contracted to reduce/eliminate smoking by [hypnosis, the patch, nicotine gum, talking to MD about medication/methods of smoking cessation]. • Pt contracted to reduce/eliminate alcohol intake. • Pt agreed to set up scheduled times for meals. • Gave pt pamphlets/literature regarding [medical condition] and interactions with [alcohol, smoking, emotional problem].

The Checklist

Checklists aren't that much different from compiling an individualized narrative list. The therapist checks off what is present, and hopefully there is a place for the therapist to list whatever symptoms the patient is experiencing but which the OTR developer did not include. As more and more managed behavioral care companies transition to computer-scannable OTR forms, checklists are going to be seen more often.

Don't agonize over whether to check the box. It's like the instructions patients are given when taking the Meyers-Briggs, the MMPI, or other similar inventories: just check whichever answer best describes, and go with your first instinct. Therapists often waste precious time over these checklists:

"Hmmmm . . . I don't know what to do. The patient's depressed mood is controlled by medication, but he or she would certainly get depressed again if he or she were to stop taking it. Do I mark 'depressed'?"

Tips for filling out symptom checklists:

- Don't make changes to the form in any way. If the form is computer-scored, altering it could mean that the computer will reject it, thus complicating and slowing down the re-certification process.
- Don't qualify choices. Therapists will draw arrows and write in "mild," "severe," and so on. Don't bother. In addition to the likelihood of computer rejection, if the managed care company had wanted that extra information, they would have used a Likert rating scale instead.
- If the patient is on medication, try to assess whether or not 95 percent to 100 percent of each symptom is gone as a result of being on the medication. If the symptom isn't almost entirely gone, mark it, regardless of medication status.

Likert-Type Rating Scale

Some therapists prefer the Likert-type rating scales, since there is the opportunity to qualify the intensity of the symptoms. However, to others, the Likert symptom rating scales are an annoyance. How does one

Assessment of the degree or intensity of symptoms is subjective.

know whether to rate a client as "mild," "moderate," "severe," and so on? It's certainly a drawback of the Likert-type rating scales that assessment of the degree or intensity of symptoms is subjective. Tips for completing a Likert-type symptom rating scale:

- Don't alter the form due to the risk of computer rejection. This will make for re-authorization hassles.
- Don't write comments on the side; a scanning computer will either ignore them or reject the form.

Choose between "mild," "moderate," and "severe" based on how this patient would compare on this symptom dimension with someone who could be considered "normal" or "un-impaired."

- Choose between "mild," "moderate," and "severe" based on how this patient would compare on this symptom dimension with someone who could be considered "normal" or "un-impaired." How close to the "un-impaired" state is the client?
- Don't debate; go with first instinct. Time spent debating between "mild" and "moderate" is time wasted. Debating neither makes the choice easier nor ends up clarifying the degree of impairment which characterizes "mild," "moderate," and so on.

Practitioner confidence in the reliability/accuracy of Likert scales could be vastly improved if managed care companies published scoring instructions, to give the therapist some rough guidelines for what constitutes "mild," "moderate," and so forth.

Social Withdrawal

- Check "Mild" if the patient reports a slight decrease in enjoyment of or engagement in interpersonal activities from the level that is normal for the patient. "Mild" social withdrawal typically does not interfere with functioning either at work or in the family.
- Check "Moderate" to indicate isolation more pronounced than at a "mild" level. "Moderate" withdrawal is more likely to be commented on by the patient's family and friends, and be a cause for concern. It may impair the patient's work/family functioning to some degree.
- Check "Severe" for complete withdrawal and rejection of social contact, to a degree which significantly impairs the patient's ability to work, function in his or her family, or perform other activities of daily living.

The Ultimate Expert

No matter the system or the form, rating symptoms is always going to be somewhat of a therapist judgment call. Aside from the patient and the patient's spouse/family, the therapist is the only person who can make a valid assessment of impairment, functioning, or symptom intensity. Regardless of their statistics, normative symptom profiles, and so forth, the managed care company is never in a position to say that a therapist is "wrong."

No matter the system or the form, rating symptoms is always going to be somewhat of a therapist judgment call.

10

Completing the OTR: Writing Treatment Plans

Chapter 9 was the prelude to the actual treatment plan, which requires the therapist to specify and describe problems, goals, interventions, and/or outcomes. Next to the symptom profile, this treatment plan component is what gets the most attention from case managers.

Choosing the Problem Areas to Highlight

In general, the component elements of managed care treatment plans are much like the hospital ones that JCAHO has required for many years:

- *Problem:* A general statement of the area being addressed in the therapy.
- *Goal:* Specifically, what is the client striving to change or achieve?
- *Intervention:* What does the therapist do to help the client achieve the goal?
- *Outcome:* The expected result of the intervention. How will the therapist be able to identify that change has taken place?

Managed care companies, fortunately, don't require a master problem list, a statement of each and every issue, even those not being actively treated. Some forms do not require any elaboration of the problems at all; instead, the treatment plan section begins with goals, conceptualizing all the preceding material as the statement of problems.

However, there are always several potential areas of focus in therapy. It is much easier to write effective goals if the client's problem areas are prioritized first. To increase the chances that the written treatment report will "pass muster," the first problem and its associated goal(s) listed should always be based on the Axis I diagnosis and the symptoms/ impairments in functioning which have led to the patient being given this diagnosis. Managed care companies may become suspicious and begin to inquire "What are you really treating?" if the treatment plan's problems and goals don't follow directly from the elements of "medical necessity" (see Chapter 7).

Other Rules of the Road When Choosing Problem Areas

Choose problems/goals that are achievable though psychotherapy (see Chapter 7). Indicating as a goal that the client will find a job, a place to live, graduate from high school/college, obtain a divorce, and so on, places the therapist at risk for being told that he or she is merely providing support that is not medically necessary.

The managed behavioral care companies also expect to see "realistic" problems and goals; however, "realistic" in the managed care world view doesn't generally refer to the overall level of possibility, but instead refers to what is achievable within a time-limited course of psychotherapy. Goals that are unlikely to be achieved within 6 or 9 months should be avoided—or narrowed in focus—on managed care treatment reports. It's also appropriate to give greater emphasis to the problems that are the most urgent to the client, and/or those problems (active substance abuse is a good example) which, by definition, must be resolved before others can successfully be addressed.

Wording the Goals

Hate writing treatment plans? Table 10.1 provides a quick reference when writing treatment reports. Additionally, there are books and software programs available to help with this task. Anything is more helpful than staring at a blank form, wondering what to write (and thinking for the umpteenth time how awful managed care is).

Behaviorally-specific goals are written in such a way that progress will be easy to demonstrate (Table 10.2). If the reader of the treatment report is able to identify what will be the observable and measurable nature of the progress the client is expected to make, then the goal is behaviorally specific.

The first problem and its associated goal(s) listed should always be based on the Axis I diagnosis and the symptoms/ impairments in functioning which have led to the patient being given this diagnosis.

Goals that are unlikely to be achieved within 6 or 9 months should be avoided—or narrowed in focus—on managed care treatment reports.

Table 10.1
"Managed Care Friendly" Goals for Various Problem Areas

Diagnosis/ Problem Area	General Goals Expected by Managed Care	Suggested Wording of Behaviorally Specific Goal(s)
ADD/ADHD	1. Use behavioral management techniques.	1. Client [patient] and parents to develop behavioral management plan, building in rewards and break periods on frequent basis. Report following plan [every weekday].
	2. Attend CHADD support group.	2. Client [patient] to call national CHADD line to find local chapter; client [patient] [and parents] to attend at least [3] meetings.
	3. Use concentration and organization techniques.	3. Client [patient] to report using concentration, focusing and organizational techniques taught in session at least [once daily].
	4. Obtain medical evaluation.	4. Client [patient] to make appointment for evaluation by pediatrician/PCP/psychiatrist.
	5. Medication compliance (if meds are prescribed).	5. Client [patient] will take medications [daily] as prescribed by MD; will use daily medication reminder case as needed.
Anger Management	1. Cognitive/behavioral and coping skills.	1. Client [patient] will report using the cognitive/behavioral and coping skills taught in session at least once [daily].
	2. Fewer anger outbursts/ no episodes of violence.	2. Client [patient] will report fewer and less intense episodes of verbal anger outbursts [not more than one hour per day], and no actual physical aggressiveness; therapist will confirm with family member, if possible.
	3. No homicidal ideation/ intent to harm others.	3. Client [patient] will report no instances of thinking about, fantasizing, or planning homicide or violence toward others.
	4. Recognize triggers of anger.	4. Client [patient] will identify, verbalize and list in writing the situations and/or people that arouse anger.
	5. Remove firearms/ safety plan.	5. Client [patient] will surrender any firearms to police [therapist, friend, etc.]; client [patient] will agree to page therapist if having ideas of harming self/others.
Anorexia	1. Minimum daily caloric intake and/or minimum daily weight; no purging.	1. Client [patient] [parents] will report [daily] adherence to meal plan, minimum [daily] caloric intake with no purging; [daily] weight will remain stable at [# lbs].
	2. Family involvement in treatment.	2. Client [patient]'s family will participate in [weekly] family sessions; family to help client maintain [daily] meal plan/caloric intake without purging.
	3. Medication compliance (if meds are prescribed).	3. Client [patient] will take medications [daily] as prescribed by MD; will use [daily] medication reminder case as needed.
	4. Obtain medical evaluation.	4. Client [patient] will obtain medical evaluation and all necessary tests related to possible malnutrition, electrolyte imbalance, etc.
	5. Obtain regular nutritional consultation/ meal plan.	5. Client [patient] will obtain nutritional evaluation; attend all follow-up appointments with nutritionist; will follow meal plan; therapist and nutritionist to consult on a regular basis.
	6. Recognize distortions in body image.	6. Client [patient] will verbalize acceptance of body size and shape; will report practicing cognitive-behavioral reframing skills on a [daily] basis.

Table 10.1 (Continued)

Diagnosis/ Problem Area	General Goals Expected by Managed Care	Suggested Wording of Behaviorally Specific Goal(s)
Biopolar Disorder	1. Medication compliance.	1. Client [patient] will take medications [daily] as prescribed by MD; will use daily medication reminder case as needed.
	2. Ongoing medication management/ coordination.	2. Client [patient] will attend all psychiatrist appointments; therapist and psychiatrist to consult at least [once monthly] and prn.
	3. Psychoeducation.	3. Client [patient] to verbalize understanding of nature of bipolar disorder; client to read pamphlets about bipolar disorder and attend at least [#] support group(s) sponsored by NAMI and/or DMDA.
	4. Recognize signs and triggers of potential manic or depressive episode.	4. Client [patient] will [daily] monitor sleep cycle, eating patterns, will exercise regularly, will refrain from using drugs/alcohol, and will inform psychiatrist immediately if signs indicate impeding manic or depressive episode.
	5. No suicidal ideation or plan.	5. [See Depression].
Bulimia	1. Family involvement in treatment.	1. [See Anorexia].
	2. Medical evaluation.	2. Client [patient] will obtain medical evaluation.
	3. Medication compliance (if meds are prescribed).	3. Client [patient] will take medications [daily] as prescribed by MD; will use daily medication reminder case as needed.
	4. Eliminate use of laxatives, diuretics, diet pills.	4. Client [patient] [parents; family] will report no use of laxatives, diuretics, and/or diet pills; family to monitor on [daily] basis.
	5. Report no binge eating or purging.	5. Client [patient] will report no binge eating or purging; will report using binge/purge prevention strategies taught in session [daily] and prn.
	6. Obtain regular nutritional consultation/ meal plan.	6. Client [patient] will obtain nutritional evaluation; attend all follow-up appointments with nutritionist; will follow meal plan; therapist and nutritionist to consult on [monthly] basis and prn.
Conduct Disorder	1. Coordination (with school, law enforcement, etc.)	1. Client [patient] [parent(s)] to sign releases of information to allow therapist to coordinate treatment with other professionals, law enforcement, and communtiy agencies. Therapist to maintain at least [bi-monthly] contact with above sources of information regarding the patient's behavior.
	2. Family involvement in treatment.	2. Client [patient]'s family to attend [weekly] therapy sessions; family to maintain [daily] behavioral program of natural consequences; parents to attend at least [weekly] meetings of support group Tough Love.
	3. Natural consequences.	3. Client [patient]'s family to [daily] enforce natural consequences of client's actions; therapist to work with school [etc.] such that client experiences natural consequences of his/her behavior in other settings as needed.
	4. Responsibility for actions.	4. Client [patient] to verbalize understanding that his/her behavior has consequences at least [twice] per session; family to report that patient refrains from blaming others for situations at least [twice per week].

Table 10.1 (Continued)

Diagnosis/ Problem Area	General Goals Expected by Managed Care	Suggested Wording of Behaviorally Specific Goal(s)
Depression	1. Cognitive/behavioral and coping skills.	1. Client [patient] will report use of cognitive-behavioral skills such as reframing at least [1x/day]; will demonstrate use of same at least [once] per session.
	2. Decreased irritability, tearfulness, anxiety, overeating.	2. Client [patient] to report episodes of tearfulness, irritability, anxiety, or overeating no more than [1x/week] each with duration no longer than [one hour].
	3. Improved mood, sleep, concentration, social contacts.	3. Client [patient] to report sad mood no more than [1x/day]; report sleeping [at least 6 hours/night 5 nights/week]; report ability to concentrate at work [at least 6 hrs/day]; report at least [1] non-work social activity per [week].
	4. Medication compliance (if meds are prescribed).	4. Client [patient] will take medications [daily] as prescribed by MD; will use [daily] medication reminder case as needed.
	5. Regulation of appetite.	5. Client [patient] will report eating 3 balanced meals per [day].
	6. No suicidal ideation or plan.	6. Client [patient] will report [at each session] the absence of suicidal thoughts or plan; will relinquish all firearms to trusted family member; agrees to page therapist before acting out any thoughts of self-harm.
Domestic Violence	1. Community resources.	1. Client [patient] will attend community support group at least [3 times]; keep on his/her person [at all times] the numbers of hotlines and safe houses.
	2. Education.	2. Client [patient] will be able to verbalize [at least 1x/session] that s/he is not at fault for partner's episodes of physical abusiveness.
	3. Empowerment.	3. Client [patient] will learn to identify assertiveness skills in session and report practicing same at least [1x/day].
	4. Protective orders/using the police.	4. Client [patient] will contact police in the event of physical abusiveness by partner and will obtain/follow through with restraining order.
	5. Remove firearms from house.	5. Client [patient] will secretly remove all firearms from the house and give to friend/family member for safekeeping.
Generalized Anxiety	1. Cognitive/behavioral and coping skills.	1. Client [patient] to report using cognitive-behavioral skills such as reframing and coping skills such as "time-out" [on daily basis, as needed].
	2. Decreased agitation, irritability, ruminating thoughts.	2. Client [patient] to display normal mental status in sessions; client to report no more than [one hour/day] of agitation, irritability, racing or ruminating thoughts.
	3. Medical evaluation.	3. Client [patient] to make appointment with PCP/medical specialist to rule out physical causes of anxiety/panic attacks.
	4. Medication compliance (if meds are prescribed).	4. Client [patient] will take medications [daily] as prescribed by MD; will use [daily] medication reminder case as needed.
	5. Relaxation.	5. Client [patient] will report practicing guided imagery/relaxation/meditation skills [2x/daily] as taught in sessions.

Table 10.1 (Continued)

Diagnosis/ Problem Area	General Goals Expected by Managed Care	Suggested Wording of Behaviorally Specific Goal(s)
Obsessive-Compulsive Disorder	1. Ability to complete daily tasks (ADLs, work/school, etc.)	1. Client [patient] to report that ADL's [specify which] are completed [on daily basis] without being slowed by OCD rituals such as handwashing, checking, etc.
	2. Decrease frequency/intensity of rituals.	2. Client [patient] to report [spouse/parents to confirm] that rituals last no longer than [30 minutes] and are no more frequent than [3 times/week].
	3. Medication compliance (if meds are prescribed).	3. Client [patient] will take medications [daily] as prescribed by MD; will use [daily] medication reminder case as needed.
	4. Cognitive/behavioral and coping skills.	4. Client [patient] to report using cognitive-behavioral skills such as reframing, examining fears for rationality/realism, and coping skills such as "time-out" [on a daily basis, as needed].
Panic Disorder	1. Ability to leave home for daily tasks (if agoraphobic).	1. Client [patient] will report leaving home [at least 1x daily] for necessary tasks such as grocery shopping, work, etc.
	2. Medical evaluation.	2. Client [patient] to make appointment with PCP/medical specialist to rule out physical causes of anxiety/panic attacks.
	3. Medication compliance (if meds are prescribed).	3. Client [patient] will take medications [daily] as prescribed by MD; will use [daily] medication reminder case as needed.
	4. Reduction in frequency and intensity of panic attacks.	4. Client [patient] will report reduction in number of panic attacks to [not more than 2x/week], and will report reduction in panic attack intensity as evidenced by length of attack [less than 5 minutes].
	5. Relaxation.	5. [See Generalized Anxiety].
Paranoia	1. Medication compliance (if meds are prescribed).	1. Client [patient] will take medications [daily] as prescribed by MD; will use [daily] medication reminder case as needed.
	2. Decrease in paranoia.	2. Client [patient] to show decreased paranoia as evidenced by behavior in sessions that is not characterized by suspicion or guardedness. Client [patient]'s family to report paranoid behavior no more than [once/month]. Client [patient] to report absence of thoughts of persecution, being watched, etc., on [daily basis].
	3. Ongoing medication management/ coordination.	3. Client [patient] will attend all psychiatrist apointments; therapist and psychiatrist to consult at least [once monthly] and prn.
Post-Traumatic Stress	1. Decrease in frequency/intensity of symptoms of hypervigilance and anxiety.	1. Client [patient] to report nightmares [not more than once per week], report episodes of panic attacks, trembling, choking, sweating, intrusive recollections, de-realization, etc. [specify symptoms] to be of shorter duration and not more frequent than [once per week]. Client to appear less agitated in sessions.
	2. Desensitization to stimuli which recall the original trauma.	2. Client [patient] to report [at least weekly] use of relaxation and self-soothing techniques paired with stimuli which are reminders of original trauma.
	3. Medication compliance (if meds are prescribed).	3. Client [patient] will take medications [daily] as prescribed by MD; will use [daily] medication reminder case as needed.

Table 10.1 (Continued)

Diagnosis/ Problem Area	General Goals Expected by Managed Care	Suggested Wording of Behaviorally Specific Goal(s)
Social Phobia	1. Cognitive/behavioral and coping skills.	1. Client [patient] will verbalize understanding of negative self-talk and messages regarding his/her "performance" in social situations; will practice reframing and identifying irrational thoughts [daily].
	2. Desensitization.	2. Client [patient] to report [at least weekly] use of relaxation techniques paired with social situations and/or contemplation of social situations.
	3. Increase social contacts.	3. Client [patient] to report a social contact at least [1x/week] outside of work.
	4. Feel more confident in social situations.	4. Client [patient] to feel more confident in social situations a.e.b. demonstration of increased eye contact in sessions; firmer handshake; calm demeanor and voice. Client to report at least one of same at each other social contact and report subjective feeling of increased confidence.
Substance Abuse/ Dependence (alcohol, prescription and/or illicit drugs)	1. Attend AA/12-Step self-help groups.	1. Client [patient] to attend at least [3] AA [NA, RR, etc.] meetings per [week], and obtain a sponsor. Report step work on [daily] basis.
	2. Develop relapse prevention plan.	2. Client [patient] to write list of triggers to drinking/using and behavioral alternatives to use instead; give list to sponsor and family members.
	3. Develop sober social support system.	3. Client [patient] to attend at least [#] social events per [month] where there is no drinking or using/sponsored by AA/NA/recovery community.
	4. Family involvement in treatment and recovery.	4. Family will attend Al-Anon and/or family sessions [weekly]; participate in relapse prevention plan; verbalize understanding of disease of alcoholism/addiction and effects on family functioning.
	5. Maintain abstinence/ sobriety.	5. Client [patient] will report [daily] abstinence from alcoholic beverages and all mood-altering drugs. Will report daily abstinence from using triggers such as [list] and [daily] abstinence from all mood-altering substances. Will verbalize understanding of cross-tolerance.
	6. Verbalize understanding of alcoholism/drug addiction as a disease.	6. Client [patient] will verbalize progressive and disease nature of alcoholism/addiction; client [patient] will read [give title of book/pamphlet].

The goals in the left-hand column of Table 10.2 are wordy and cumbersome, aren't they? But they're what managed care wants—even though their forms give little room to word the goals! It would be easier to be able to say:

- Client to reduce depression.
- Client to be less anxious.

Table 10.2
The Relationships between Goals, Progress, and Identifying Progress

Goal ────────────▶	Progress Indicators ──────────▶	Identifying Progress
Client to report lowered levels of depressive symptoms, i.e., brighter mood, less tearfulness, able to go to sleep/stay asleep, less irritable, no suicidal ideation, able to concentrate, taking pleasure in activities, engaging in social contacts.	Happier mood; concentration Reduced tearfulness; irritability Sleep—quality and quantity Taking pleasure in activities; Social activities.	Client self-report Scores on BDI or other inventory/checklist Behavior observable in session Collateral reports from family/friends Reports from other professionals involved
Client to report no more than 1 panic attack per month. Client to report panic attacks of decreased duration.	Duration and frequency of panic attacks.	Client self-report; reports by family/friends Reports from other professionals involved Log/journal duration of each panic attack
Patient to report ability to manage anxiety on a daily basis through the use of relaxation, meditation, cognitive reframing techniques.	Use of techniques to manage anxiety, such as relaxation, meditation, thought-stopping, etc.	Client self-report; observation in sessions Assessments of other professionals Anxiety checklists/measurement inventories
Client to verbally commit to plan to maintain abstinence from alcohol/drugs which includes 4 12-step meetings per week; contact with sponsor on a daily basis; weekly aftercare group; and family therapy.	Attendance at 12-step meetings; contact with sponsor; abstinence; collateral interviews with family; aftercare participation.	Self-Report; observation in session of behavior and appearance; info from other professionals; urine drug screen; 12-step attendance sheet and/or meeting journal
Client to report allowing self to grieve by remembering spouse and talking about him.	Photo albums; journal; talk to family/friends; support group.	Self-report; observation in session; collateral info from family/friends
Patient to weigh self not more than once daily; exercise not more than 45 minutes daily; consume 1,000 calories daily; make at least one positive self-statement about body per session.	Frequency of weighing self, exercise, and positive/negative statements about body; daily caloric intake.	Self-report; observation in session; collateral info from family; coordination with other professionals involved; daily caloric intake log/other measurement tool

- Client to stop abuse of alcohol/drugs.
- Client to grieve death of spouse.
- Client to overcome anorexia.

Consistently, outpatient case managers who were interviewed mentioned that after hostile behavior, the next thing most likely to make them remember therapists' names for a negative reason was poor treatment plans. And the case managers, when they said poor treatment plan, almost always clarified that they meant lack of specific goals and outcome/progress criteria.

"I don't do this, and I never have problems getting re-authorization." Treatment plans with nonspecific goals are often approved. The temptation for an overworked case manager is to think, "I know what Dr. Jones means, I'll just approve it and save myself the phone call." Particularly when clients obviously meet other criteria for medical necessity, such as serious symptoms, one or more risk factors, or when there haven't been high numbers of sessions previously authorized, the case manager might not bother to call for clarification.

A very common case manager response to vague treatment goals is to authorize only a few more sessions, usually just enough to cover ongoing treatment while the therapist fills out a new OTR or schedules a telephone review.

But is the number of sessions they authorize at one time shrinking? A very common case manager response to vague treatment goals is to authorize only a few more sessions, usually just enough to cover ongoing treatment while the therapist fills out a new OTR or schedules a telephone review. Since there are some companies and accounts who will only authorize 5 or fewer sessions at any one time to begin with, it's hard to be sure what a skimpy certification means without calling the case manager and asking why. It may be worth experimenting with writing behaviorally-specific goals, to see if the number of sessions authorized at one time increases.

How specific is specific enough? The trick to writing behaviorally specific goals is to put symptoms in reverse. Start with the identified symptoms or problems in functioning, rather than making a global statement about the diagnosis improving. Then identify: (1) what needs to change, or what will be different? and (2) frequency at which the change will occur or be maintained.

The easiest way to create behaviorally-specific goals is to work from the original list of symptoms, answering the question, "When the symptoms are cleared up, what will be the result?" For example, a client with depression has the following symptoms: tearfulness, suicidal ideation, can't get up in the morning, anhedonia.

1. *Tearfulness:* Report less frequent crying episodes (i.e., not more than once per week), report less intense/shorter crying episodes.
2. *Suicidal ideation:* Report no suicidal ideation or plan; will not act on ideas.
3. *Can't get up in the* A.M.*:* Report getting up when alarm rings each weekday.
4. *Anhedonia:* Report taking pleasure in at least one activity per (time unit).

Indicating a frequency for the achievement of a goal is desirable, if there is room on the form, because it increases the specificity of the outcome measurement. Listing frequency of goal achievement may actually be a way to protect the client from a decision that the client has had too many sessions. If the therapist can demonstrate that the client has not yet achieved the goal to a frequency reasonable enough to prevent relapse if discharged, it is telling the case manager why sessions continue to be medically necessary.

Indicating a frequency for the achievement of a goal increases the specificity of the outcome measurement.

> Therapist Walt Skinner, PhD, was treating Alan Mandrake, who was extremely depressed following the disappearance of his wife. HPBH had authorized 40 sessions to date with Dr. Skinner. His benefit plan allowed unlimited outpatient visits as long as HPBH authorized medical necessity. Alan was also seeing Fred Sigmund, MD, for medication management. At the beginning of therapy, Alan continually expressed suicidal ideation and, although he assured Dr. Skinner that he would not actively take his own life, he acted out his suicidal ideation by driving very fast, not looking when crossing the street, standing at the very edge of the subway platform, and so on. Alan was lethargic, had formerly been athletic and worked out daily, but had stopped after the police could find no trace of his wife. He had gained about 30 pounds in the last 6 months. He had been put on probation by his boss for frequent tardiness to work, but could not make himself get up in the morning or care about the consequences to his job. He couldn't concentrate at work, and was socially isolated, rebuffing all attempts by family and friends to help him.
>
> On the next OTR, Dr. Skinner reported that the medications were helping and that Alan's symptoms had lessened, although he still needed therapy. Kay Smanager called Dr. Skinner, asking why Alan still needed to be seen

if he was doing better. Frustrated, Dr. Skinner spelled out each one of Alan's original presenting symptoms. For each symptom, Dr. Skinner indicated where Alan had been at the time treatment began, where Alan was now, and what needed to happen before discharge would be appropriate. For example, Dr. Skinner wrote:

1. Beginning of treatment: frequent (4–5 × /wk) tardiness to work due to not being able to get up in the morning.
2. Now: Still tardy to work once or twice per week.
3. When ready for discharge: Alan will report tardiness once per month or less, and boss will take him off probation in this regard.

Although Dr. Skinner privately thought this would do no good because he had already had 40 sessions, Kay responded enthusiastically and authorized another 3 months worth of sessions.

The idea is to be able to pinpoint exactly when the client is ready for discharge.

The idea is to be able to pinpoint exactly when the client is ready for discharge. With the growing trend toward outcomes measurement and utilization review by real-time outcomes (see Chapter 8), look for the powers that be at the managed care companies to increasingly pass the pressure of demonstrating outcomes onto the shoulders of mental health professionals. And, for those in a group practice with capitated contracts, "the powers that be" may not refer to the managed care company, but to committees of practice colleagues.

Measuring the Outcome

Behaviorally-specific goals include in their phrasing the indicator(s) by which it will become known the client has achieved the goal.

Behaviorally-specific goals include in their phrasing the indicator(s) by which it will become known the client has achieved the goal. It is clear from Dr. Skinner's report exactly when Alan will have met his treatment goal. The means of knowing (client self-report, in Alan's case) will also be clear from the wording. Client self-report is the most common way of knowing when goals will be achieved.

What else is there, besides self-report? Consider using one of these options, if appropriate to the circumstances:

- "Client will demonstrate to therapist in sessions that . . ."
- Report from a spouse/significant other.
- Report from a parent/other family member.
- Report from another professional involved with the client (teacher, primary care MD, etc.).

- Improved score on a validated scale.
- External events which indicate progress (client's grades, promotion at work, decision to get married or divorced, leaves abusive marriage, Family Services grants unsupervised visitation, agrees to take antidepressant, attends AA meetings, etc.).
- Completed written relapse prevention/"alternative-behavior" plan or other therapeutic homework assignments.

A.E.B.

A QI person I once knew stressed these three words: "as evidenced by," which is another method of writing goals such that the method of measuring the outcome, as well as the outcome itself, is easily identifiable.

> Dr. Skinner wrote, "Alan will be less depressed as evidenced by self-report of reduced tearfulness (less than one episode per week)."

Remembering these three words can help in the process of writing goals. To save room on the treatment report form, "as evidenced by" can be abbreviated "a.e.b." The phrase "as evidenced by" ties the overall, nonspecific goal (reducing Alan's depression) with:

1. The means by which the therapist will know that progress has been made (self-report).
2. A measurement of how the goal will be achieved (reduced crying episodes).
3. The frequency with which the goal will be achieved (crying episodes no more than once per week).

The 3-Step Method

However the treatment plan's goals are phrased, if they are behaviorally-specific, these three elements will always be present:

1. *Target.*
2. *When ready for discharge, how frequently is the target being achieved?*
3. *Means of knowing that the target is met.*

In general, case managers expect behaviorally-specific goals with defined outcomes most when they think the client should be ready for discharge, and/or if they are feeling hard put to justify continued treatment because of the number of sessions the client has already been authorized.

Interventions can be defined as "what the therapist does with the client to help him or her move from goal to outcome."

The First Time's the Easiest

Less is expected with the first treatment report submitted, particularly if there have been only two or three sessions since the start of therapy. Therapists writing that first OTR on a client, then, can get away with goals that are less behaviorally-specific than subsequently, when there have been more sessions. In general, case managers expect behaviorally-specific goals with defined outcomes most when they think the client should be ready for discharge, and/or if they are feeling hard put to justify continued treatment because of the number of sessions the client has already been authorized.

Behaviorally-Specific Treatment Interventions

Interventions can be defined as "what the therapist does with the client to help him or her move from goal to outcome." Not all OTRs ask the therapist to specify interventions; some will infer the interventions from the goals. Interventions, in themselves, do not determine medical necessity. With only a few major exceptions (such as medication; see Chapter 11), to date managed care companies haven't paid much attention to HOW therapists and clients have achieved therapeutic goals, so long as the client could be successfully discharged within a timeframe the company perceived as "reasonable." Expect this to change, however, as managed care companies continue their move away from emphasizing "medical necessity" to instead evaluating practice in terms of treatment guidelines. Treatment guidelines, otherwise known as "best practices guidelines," are all about interventions (see Chapter 7).

Write the behaviorally-specific goals first, and the interventions will follow. The interventions should fit the goals and logically follow from them. Goals are the foundation of the house; without them, the interventions are nothing more than a loose pile of bricks. Table 10.3 demonstrates this link.

Table 10.3 was created by inserting typical interventions between the Goals and Progress Indicators columns of Table 10.2. The Interventions column primarily features techniques: communication skills teaching, identifying triggers of anxiety, and so forth. Just listing such techniques will rank a treatment report among the best; many therapists simply indicate "individual therapy," "marital therapy," and so on when OTR

Table 10.3
The Relationships between Goals, Interventions and Progress

Goal ⟶	Interventions ⟶	Progress Indicators
Client to report lowered levels of depressive symptoms, i.e., brighter mood, less tearfulness, able to go to sleep/stay asleep, less irritable, no suicidal ideation, able to concentrate, taking pleasure in activities, engaging in social contacts.	Refer for psychopharmacological evaluation; help client identify and monitor sympotoms; set schedule of pleasurable/social activities; teach sleep hygiene	Happier mood; concentration Reduced tearfulness; irritability Sleep-quality and quantity Taking pleasure in activities Social activities
Client to report no more than 1 panic attack per month. Client to report panic attacks of decreased duration.	Identify thoughts/situations which trigger panic attacks; teach and practice deep breathing	Duration and frequency of panic attacks
Patient to report ability to manage anxiety on a daily basis through the use of relaxation, meditation, cognitive reframing techniques.	Psychopharmacological evaluation Teach relaxation and meditation Teach and practice cognitive reframing	Use of techniques to manage anxiety
Client to verbally commit to plan to maintain abstinence from alcohol/drugs which includes 4 12-step meetings per week; contact with sponsor on a daily basis; weekly aftercare group; and family therapy.	Education on recovery, family disease, 12-step work; confront "using" beliefs; regular collateral family contact; urine/breath tests	Attendance at 12-step meetings; contact with sponsor; abstinence; collateral interviews with family; aftercare participation
Client to report allowing self to grieve by remembering spouse and talking about him.	Normalize need to share memories; encourage and support	Photo albums; journal; talk to family/friends; support group
Patient to weigh self not more than once daily; exercise not more than 45 minutes daily; consume 1,000 calories daily; make at least one positive self-statement about body per session.	Refer to dietician for meal planning; regular contacts with family/other; professionals; teach and practice cognitive-behavioral techniques	Frequency of weighing self, exercise, and positive/negative statements about body; daily caloric intake

forms ask for interventions. But there's another way of being even more behaviorally-specific.

Verbs, Verbs, Verbs

Verbs connote action and are a great way to show how the therapist's actions can help the client achieve the desired outcome(s).

Use verbs such as *teach, practice, show, guide, facilitate, demonstrate, confront, suggest, recommend, role-play, identify, develop,* and *educate.* Verbs connote action and are a great way to show how the therapist's actions can help the client achieve the desired outcome(s). Assuming there is room to do so on the form, include the verbs, as opposed to just listing a technique or theoretical orientation.

"Cognitive-behavioral therapy," for example, can be transformed from a general therapeutic modality to a set of more behaviorally-specific interventions.

- *Teach* client to *identify* irrational thoughts which promote feelings of sadness, worthlessness, or anxiety.
- *Confront* client's self-deprecating statements and *show him or her* how these promote his or her feelings of sadness, worthlessness, anxiety.

Verbs can transform a technique such as "communication skills" into:

- *Demonstrate* active listening.
- *Practice* making "I" statements to use during conflicts with spouse.

Intervention "Do's and Don'ts"

Community Resources and Self-Help Groups

A common misconception is that therapists should only include support groups if the client is actually going, or has agreed to go.

Managed care companies love documentation of referrals to community support groups. Any mention of substance abuse, in particular, almost automatically carries with it the expectation of a referral to one or more 12-step groups (see Chapter 11).

For the purposes of an outpatient treatment report, it's best to document mentioning relevant support groups and/or community resources to the client, assuming this has been done. A common misconception is that therapists should only include support groups if the client is actually going, or has agreed to go. Not true. If a therapist says to a client, "Have you considered Al-Anon?" or "Do you know about CHADD?," that's an intervention. The client may disagree or may not follow through, but that doesn't mean the therapist never intervened.

Some therapists believe that mentioning a community resource or support group means that managed care will deny sessions, because there's the community resource out there which the company doesn't have to pay for. I can say honestly that I've never personally encountered this. Community resources or self-help/support groups aren't a direct substitute for therapy, only an adjunct to it.

Therapeutic Homework

Managed care companies love it. Although it may be helpful to specify the nature of the homework, even just writing "therapeutic homework" in the list of interventions can be helpful.

Avoid Using Buzz Words

Use of *buzz words*, terms therapists think managed care wants to hear, can work both for or against a therapist, depending on how they are used. I often saw treatment reports like this:

> *Goal:* Reduce depression.
> *Interventions:* Cognitive-behavioral.

This sort of answer doesn't impress case managers. Quite the opposite, in fact. It tells them nothing, at best, and may look passive-aggressive at worst. For the sake of the client's getting authorization, the therapist would look better if he or she said (or wrote):

- "Teach reframing of negative attributions."
- "Identify irrational beliefs such as the need for perfection."
- "Confront client's personalization of events."
- "Identify all or nothing thinking."

Even something as generic as "Cognitive-behavioral approach to identifying triggers of depression and developing positive self-talk" is usually good enough.

Progress

The Catch-22 Factor

When writing treatment plans, it's always a balancing act with regard to the client's progress. If the therapist is too enthusiastic about the client's progress, the case manager might get the wrong idea and conclude there is no longer a need for therapy. On the other hand, the treatment report must show that the client is achieving some benefit. It's a clause common to most medical necessity codes that clients must be achieving benefit (or be able to achieve benefit) in order for continued therapy to be "medically necessary" (see Chapter 7).

Reporting Progress

Progress indicators can be derived directly from the "behaviorally-specific" goals, as shown by Tables 10.2 and 10.3 which depict the relationships between the treatment plan elements. As with interventions, the nature of progress has been somewhat ignored in outpatient utilization review. The current push toward demonstrable outcomes will increase the pressure to frame progress in much the same behaviorally-specific way as the other treatment plan elements.

If the goals have been written in a behaviorally-specific manner, and particularly if a target frequency has been established, then reporting progress is simply a mechanical matter of indicating whether or not the client has achieved the goal, and to what extent. Dr. Skinner's report on his client, Alan, is a good example of how to report partial progress in this framework. Other examples:

- Patient began treatment reporting crying episodes daily. Is now reporting tearfulness only three or four times weekly.
- Client reports that panic attacks are still daily, but that he is able to calm himself down somewhat more quickly, after only ten minutes as opposed to a half hour or so.

Progress Rating Scales

Sometimes outpatient treatment reports feature Likert-type rating scales for the client's progress, similar to the rating scales used for severity and presence of symptoms. Other companies' forms will request therapists to estimate the percentage of the goal achieved. As with rating symptoms, this is generally a difficult task for therapists, because "progress" is a process, not a discrete event. For instance, clients may verbalize awareness of their issues relatively early in therapy, but actual behavior change lags behind. So does that get a 1, indicating "mild" progress, or a 2, meaning "moderate" progress? Don't sweat it.

When therapists do not report even small degrees of progress as a result of 10 to 20 sessions of therapy, there is a risk that the managed care company will become more directive of treatment, under the guise of "it's not working, let's do (or add) something else." The conclusion that *"it's not working,"* may or may not be true, depending on the individual client's situation, just as changing the treatment plan may or may not be clinically appropriate. Managed care companies rarely deny further sessions outright when a client is not making progress that they consider fast enough; instead, the most common approach is that of a directive for the client to seek medication (see Chapter 11). Therapists can best help their clients obtain continued authorization and reduce the risk of interference by finding some indicator(s) of progress, however small. In this respect, forms that ask for a narrative description of progress might be somewhat easier to complete. It's okay to say things like:

Therapists can best help their clients obtain continued authorization and reduce the risk of interference by finding some indicator(s) of progress, however small.

- "Patient is less guarded in sessions."
- "Patient shares feelings in sessions."
- "Client actively participates in sessions." (More behavioral than saying "patient is motivated.")
- "Patient is making better eye contact."
- "Client verbalizes awareness that he needs to take responsibility for controlling his anger."

Unless the patient is truly going to need long-term therapy, it's generally a good idea to reserve these sorts of statements about very slight progress to the first or second treatment report. Case managers seeing these sorts of comments after 20 sessions are probably going to call the therapist.

If the case manager does call to raise the issue of "lack of progress" (and to direct treatment that's "not working"), be able to provide well-reasoned, clinical answers to these questions:

1. Identify any obstacles that appear to be blocking the pace of the client's progress.

2. What specifically needs to change regarding these obstacles if the client is to eventually achieve the goal(s)?

3. Are 1 and 2 changeable via psychotherapy?

4. How much time will this process be estimated to take?

5. [if therapist disagrees with case manager's recommendation of treatment plan modifications] Explain why these modifications would be counter-therapeutic or ineffective.

Discharge Plan

Setting a Date

Stay general, and never give a date more than 3 or 4 months beyond the date of the treatment plan.

Discharge plans are a requirement for inpatient treatment teams, but not many OTR forms ask for anything beyond an estimated date of discharge. Stay general, and never give a date more than 3 or 4 months beyond the date of the treatment plan. Therapists who indicate a date (no matter how honest or realistic) of a year or two down the road look as if they want to keep the patient in therapy forever. The way to go is to repeatedly give 3 to 4 month timeframes and then on each treatment report identify current symptoms, impairments, and goals that meet medical necessity criteria.

For patients that truly do require more than 20 or 30 sessions, look at it the way managed care does: goals listed on a current treatment report are the primary goals for the next 3 months. At the next treatment report, the goals and interventions have been altered based on circumstances and/or progress, and are now "new" goals and interventions, which will be the primary focus of therapy for another 3 months. And so on.

Narrative Discharge Plan

If required by the OTR form to write a discharge plan (this is rare), tie it directly to the goals that were listed for the client. It's best to write no more than one sentence, answering the question "What kind of progress will the client be exhibiting when he or she is ready to terminate?"

Two pointers when answering a question about discharge planning:

1. Always refer to achievement of the goals "as listed above."

2. State that the plan is to gradually reduce the frequency of sessions, also known as titration.

Managed care likes treatment plans where clients are being seen less frequently than once per week. *"Continued sessions spaced farther apart will allow client the opportunity to refine and maintain skills learned in therapy, and will support effective termination and relapse prevention"* is an effective way to phrase titration of sessions.

Writing Managed Care Treatment Plans for Long-Term Clients

Yes, there are still such clients; even in managed care. For those whose outpatient benefits aren't limited to 20 or 30 sessions per year, at any rate.

Although case managers will of course expect to see some semblance of "behaviorally-specific" goals on all OTRs, watch out for narrowing the focus too much with clients who aren't good candidates for "brief solution-focused therapy." Let's face it; teaching problem-solving, cognitive-behavioral, interpersonal communication, assertiveness skills, and so forth, is valuable, but the types of clients who can be successful with only 10 or 20 sessions of such "brief therapy" are generally fairly high-functioning to begin with. There are many patients with multiple issues and/or serious disorders for whom "brief solution-focused" treatment is nothing more than a Band-Aid. Good case managers know this.

Recall the case of Rose Jones, from Chapter 7. Rose was a 60-year-old woman with multiple issues of anxiety, agoraphobia, depression, chronic pain, compulsive overeating, obesity, and a past history of sexual abuse by her father. The progress of a client like Rose is likely to be very slow and in small increments. Nor is she going to have the ability to first meet one goal, then tackle the next, and so on. Narrowing the focus (i.e., choosing only one or two problem areas and goals to work on) for a client with several highly interrelated and chronic issues will risk the managed care company thinking that he or she can complete treatment in fewer sessions than is realistic. It's a lot of work in the beginning, but listing each and every problem area may be necessary to get it "on the record" that this client may need longer-term treatment.

If the client's problems are very severe, point out the many obstacles to faster progress. For clients who have already had large numbers of sessions authorized, identifying obstacles to progress—or how far the client really has to go—is vital in order to help the case manager understand why sessions should continue to be authorized.

Narrowing the focus (i.e., choosing only one or two problem areas and goals to work on) for a client with several highly interrelated and chronic issues will risk the managed care company thinking that he or she can complete treatment in fewer sessions than is realistic.

Clients Who Require Long-Term Supportive or "Maintenance" Therapy

Be on the lookout for the number of administrative hoops to multiply, and the number of sessions to be authorized per treatment report to drop, with a "mental health parity" client, particularly if the benefit is administered by a for-profit entity.

The mental health parity movement is beginning to protect the rights of clients with serious mental illness, and clients living in states with tough mental health parity statutes are virtually guaranteed authorization. But there's a downside. Be on the lookout for the number of administrative hoops to multiply, and the number of sessions to be authorized per treatment report to drop, with a "mental health parity" client, particularly if the benefit is administered by a for-profit entity. Companies won't admit it, but these requirements, such as the need to send a treatment plan every three or four sessions, are financially effective because therapists and clients alike tend to give up out of sheer frustration.

On the state level, every mental health parity law is different. Many don't include substance abuse. Others don't cover clients in self-funded, ERISA plans (see Chapter 12). So take care—and do your homework—before boldly telling the managed care company that they are legally obligated to continue to pay for a client's treatment.

However, even in the absence of parity laws, managed care isn't opposed to maintenance therapy, if it keeps a client out of the hospital. The therapist's task is to convince the managed care company that the client really does need what extended supportive therapy can offer. Here are some tips:

1. *Explain the clinical reasoning behind the request for long-term supportive therapy.* "Vincent is a rapid-cycling bipolar client who requires frequent medication adjustments to maintain stability and stay out of the hospital. The consistent structure of weekly outpatient therapy is vital to helping him continue to identify and manage his symptoms, stay medication-compliant, and maintain current level of functioning."

Managed care rarely quibbles about maintenance clients being seen once or twice a month, but they may hesitate to continue to pay for weekly visits.

2. *Be sure to have a very good explanation if requesting weekly therapy.* Managed care rarely quibbles about maintenance clients being seen once or twice a month, but they may hesitate to continue to pay for weekly visits. Some, such as ValueOptions (1999) even state unequivocally in their "medical necessity" criteria that maintenance treatment is not, by definition, conducted more frequently than on a biweekly basis.

   One reason for requesting weekly sessions might be if there is reason to suspect impending decompensation. For example, periods of major medication changes when the client is tapering off the old medication and/or is building up to a therapeutic dose of the new medication, are higher-risk periods during which it may be appropriate for the client to be seen more often. Requests for weekly sessions for purposes of maintaining stabilization are likely to be granted, but only until the client is re-stabilized and the crisis has passed.

3. *Be sure to state why the client is better off continuing in individual therapy as opposed to being referred to a group.* However, since groups are often the treatment of choice for clients requiring long-term supportive therapy, expect that it may be a hard sell to convince the case manager. Some valid reasons (if true), why a referral to a group might be contra-indicated:

Be sure to state why the client is better off continuing in individual therapy as opposed to being referred to a group.

- There is no group available in the area.
- The client is significantly higher- or lower-functioning than the clients in the available group(s).
- There is co-morbid social phobia or agoraphobia.
- The client is dual-diagnosis and there are no groups available which understand and respect the needs of dual-diagnosis clients (*for example, some AA groups pressure these clients into giving up their medications*).
- Complicating personality disorder.

Always be sure to mention the more expensive alternatives of not continuing in outpatient therapy: "*Client needs continued support to maintain current level of functioning. Relapse could result in hospitalization.*" If there is not much likelihood of hospitalization, make a similar argument for the cost-effectiveness of weekly therapy in terms of maintained productivity at the workplace, improved family functioning (i.e., reducing the likelihood of other family members needing therapy), and/or reduced long-term medical costs.

Always be sure to mention the more expensive alternatives of not continuing in outpatient therapy.

What If the OTR Isn't Acceptable?

If the treatment report is unacceptable, it should never happen that the case manager simply denies further treatment (see Chapter 12). Prior to issuing a pending denial, case managers have these options:

1. Call the therapist to obtain additional information for the formal justification.
2. Ask an assistant to call the therapist to obtain the additional information.
3. Send the OTR back to the therapist with a written note indicating what needs to be completed before authorization will take place.
4. Certify one or two sessions and communicate in one of the following ways what needs to be submitted to obtain more sessions:

   A note on the authorization letter.

   A voice mail message.

   A separate form letter.

Any of these, although they might not constitute a denial, are certainly annoyances to busy therapists who don't want to be bothered with managed care any more than is absolutely necessary. Taking steps to ensure OTRs "pass muster" can eliminate the risk of additional requests for information by case managers and smooth the re-authorization process.

11

Managed Care's
Clinical Predispositions

Dina Troy, LCSW, received a voice mail message from a case manager at Ultra-Care Behavioral Health, Nelson Lawrence, about her OTR for Woodrow Alan. Woody's symptoms of sadness, low self-esteem, mild anxiety, and difficulty concentrating were of long duration, and she had given him the diagnosis of Dysthymia. Dina had seen him about 15 times. The message indicated that Woody should be referred for psychiatric evaluation to see if medication was appropriate.

Dina had, in fact, already mentioned the possibility of medication to Woody, but he had reacted by becoming very anxious, thinking that medication meant that he was "crazy," and that Dina was giving up on him. She was currently in the process of educating Woody about the biological basis of depression, but felt that it had to be done carefully, in a way that would convey support and empowerment, not abandonment or impatience with perceived lack of progress.

Medication

Why the preference for pills? Even for disorders such as depression where brief cognitive-behavioral therapy models have been shown to be at least as effective as medication, managed care tends to favor pharmacology over psychotherapy as a "cheaper" and more quantifiable approach to symptom reduction. Certainly a large part of the reason is the medical model on which managed care is based, and our cultural preferences favoring medication. Whether or not medication is really cheaper than psychotherapy, if all factors are taken into account, is debatable. Variables include the length of psychotherapy, the length of time the patient remains on the medication, the dose of the medication, and the particular drug that is prescribed. Some psychiatric medications are quite expensive.

Managed care does tend to favor pharmacology over psychotherapy as a "cheaper" and more quantifiable approach to symptom reduction.

Paying for the Pills

But often, not all the factors are considered when determining cost. When behavioral health benefits are "carved out" from the medical benefits (see Chapter 1), it is usually the general medical portion of the plan that pays all prescription costs—even for antidepressants. The carve-out managed behavioral health plan covers only the psychiatrist visits. Since many psychotropic drugs are prescribed by primary care physicians, since psychiatrists don't always see their patients on a weekly basis, and/or are not allowed more than a 15- or 30-minute med check, the economics even more clearly favor medication. This is particularly true with contracts that are "at-risk" (see Chapter 7), because symptom reduction can quantifiably be demonstrated with less economic investment on the part of the carve-out managed behavioral health plan.

Managing the Managed Care Company if Clients Refuse Medication

Chances are good that Dina simply didn't document Woody's reaction when she mentioned medication and what her plans were with regards to educating him about depression. If the reason(s) why the client is refusing medication, or why medication is inappropriate, are clearly documented in outpatient treatment reports, chances are excellent that busy case managers will simply make a note of it and move on to the next client. Mention of any of the following circumstances with regard to medication, for clients who are not on medication, is generally sufficient to allow an OTR to pass muster:

- Client is afraid/unsure about medication, and the therapist is currently working to help educate the client about the benefits of psychotropic medication.
- A psychiatric evaluation has been scheduled/looking for a psychiatrist.
- A specific clinical rationale regarding why medication is not appropriate for this particular client.
- Client refuses to consider medication (history of poor outcomes and/or major side effects when medication previously taken should be mentioned, if applicable). If the client gives a reason for his or her refusal, document it.

- Medical conditions/other current prescriptions that contraindicate psychiatric medication, in the opinion of the client's doctor.
- Client wants to try herbal alternatives. (Yes, it is okay to mention St. John's Wort on an OTR!)
- Female client who is either pregnant, trying to get pregnant, or is breast-feeding.
- Primary care physician or psychiatrist already evaluated and was of the opinion that medication is not necessary.

Therapists who don't mention medication, even if they think it's very obvious why medication is not clinically indicated, eventually will be called by a case manager about the medication issue, and this risk increases steadily with the number of sessions previously authorized.

No Meds = No Therapy?

There are a lot of horror stories floating about featuring evil managed care companies that deny treatment because patients refuse to take medication. In reality, it's hard to distinguish from the stories whether or not these are actual denials (see Chapter 12). Although case managers are expected by their employer to make recommendations for more effective treatment, as part of the value-added service of case management, ultimately, the practitioner is the treating professional, and in the end the managed care company has only two choices: authorize as medically necessary, or issue a formal denial. If symptoms are strong enough to warrant a recommendation of medication, then by definition there's medical necessity. Clinical suggestions from case managers, even those such as Nelson's which are stated in a very directive manner, should *never* be interpreted as a threat that sessions will be denied if the suggestions are not implemented.

Clinical suggestions can be very directive in highly managed, at-risk accounts (see Chapter 7). Case managers do consciously use the tactic of authorizing just one or two more sessions, hinting strongly at a denial if the patient isn't at least in the process of getting on medication when it comes time for the next review. Another tactic is to tell the therapist that "the patient's benefit plan requires that patients with depression diagnoses be on medication." If it gets to this point, ask for a copy of the Summary Plan Description of the benefit plan, with the relevant passage highlighted. The reality is that Summary Plan Descriptions are not

Therapists who don't mention medication eventually will be called by a case manager about the medication issue, and this risk increases steadily with the number of sessions previously authorized.

If symptoms are strong enough to warrant a recommendation of medication, then by definition there's medical necessity.

usually prescriptive of treatments for given disorders because employers don't want to risk lawsuits for practicing medicine without a license. Case managers say these things because this is how the managed care company has chosen to interpret the client's benefit plan, and this is what they are instructed to do.

Expectations for Documenting Medications

Minimally, list the names of the medications the client is taking. Managed care companies expect practitioners to have not only the name of the medication, but also the information on dosages and delivery (in the A.M., twice daily, etc.). They also expect therapists to note:

- Current side effects of medication.
- The patient's level of compliance with medication.
- Effectiveness of medication as reported by the client.
- History of poor response to medications/side effects/lack of compliance.

All of these questions may or may not be on the OTR form, but they're expected to be in the treatment record (see Table 4.2).

And even that's not all. NCQA expects coordination with primary care physicians (NCQA, 2000, QI 8.2), and to achieve accreditation, managed care companies must document and monitor therapists' coordination. To this end, there is almost always a question on OTRs asking if the therapist has consulted with the primary care physician. By definition, if there has been a consultation, the therapist will have been briefed by the medical professional about names of medical as well as psychiatric prescriptions, dosages, patient compliance, and side effects, and will have documented this information in the treatment record.

All managed care companies, particularly those with EAPs, are vehement about the need for thorough assessment of substance abuse.

Substance Abuse and 12-Step Groups

All managed care companies, particularly those with EAPs, are vehement about the need for thorough assessment of substance abuse. Why? Untreated substance abuse costs employers and health plans a great deal of money each year. Additionally, it's simple clinical common sense that undiagnosed and/or untreated substance abuse significantly lowers the chance of a positive outcome when a patient is treated for another Axis I disorder. Pressure is put on managed behavioral care organizations by purchasers to make sure that substance abuse is assessed and treated when employees use their behavioral health benefits as well as when they use the employee assistance program (EAP).

Because it's an area of such vital concern to employers, substance abuse is a popular area for financially at-risk performance guarantees (see Chapter 1). Cigna Behavioral Health (formerly MCC Behavioral Care), for example, guarantees a lower rate of absenteeism, decreased emergency room and medical/surgical inpatient utilization, reduced patient reports of depression, and improved marital/family relationships, at six months after the onset of treatment for substance-related disorders (Bengen-Seltzer, 1998).

Because it's an area of such vital concern to employers, substance abuse is a popular area for financially at-risk performance guarantees.

It always comes back to the therapist. When managed care companies make performance guarantees that are financially at-risk, pressure is put on the case managers to be sure that their documentation addresses the issues relevant to the guarantee. To document achievement of whatever is guaranteed, the case managers must get the information from either the client, or whoever is treating the client—the therapist.

Substance Abuse Assessment 101

Minimally, what do managed care companies expect from a substance abuse assessment? Quite a lot, if the client indicates drinking/using with a frequency and/or quantity great enough to suspect that there might be a problem:

- *Frequency and amount of client's use.* How often? How much? What is the client's drug of choice? Clients are not always very specific, and sometimes a bit of probing is needed.
- *Method of use.* Snorting, inhalation ("huffing"), IV use, pills, smoking?
- *Context of use.* Does the client drink/use alone? With a group of friends? Does he or she have to sneak around in order to use? How does the client obtain his or her drug of choice?
- *Age of first use/length of time used.* At what age did the client begin use of each substance? What were the circumstances of the first use? If the client doesn't remember when he or she began using, about how many years has he or she used?

- *Consequences in any life areas as a result of drug/alcohol use.* Consider several areas: job/school, legal, financial, past and present relationships, family, friends, medical.

- *Past/present unsuccessful attempts to cut down/control/quit using.* This is right out of *DSM-IV;* it's one of the criteria for a diagnosis of substance dependence (APA, 1994).

- *Previous treatment, including participation in 12-step groups.* Was the client's experience positive or negative? Did treatment or self-help work? If the client stayed abstinent, for how long? Was he or she clean and sober from all drugs, or just the drug of choice? What triggered the relapse? If the client's response to treatment was negative, was treatment made mandatory by some external person or entity?

- *Family history of substance abuse.* Try not to settle for just a yes or no answer from the client. Which family member(s) abused drugs/alcohol? Did the client interact much with the using family member(s) as a child? Did the family member(s) ever get help? Did the family member(s) stay clean/sober?

- *History/present withdrawal syndromes.* If there is a significant alcohol and/or drug history, this must be assessed. Withdrawal can cause potential medical complications or even be fatal in some cases. If there is any chance of a withdrawal syndrome, the client should immediately be referred for detox.

It does sound like a lot, but look at it this way: if the client just has the occasional martini, a glass of wine with dinner, or a beer with buddies on the weekend, most of these questions won't be relevant. But, if there is more of a problem, the rest of the questions naturally follow. You don't have to be any kind of substance abuse expert to understand why these questions need to be asked.

Shortcut: The CAGE Method

CAGE is an acronym that's been around a lot longer than managed care. It primarily refers to alcohol use. If the full list of substance abuse assessment questions seems too much of a chore, consider using the CAGE and then referring to a certified alcohol/drug professional for a more in-depth assessment if there is reason to believe the patient might have a problem. If the answer to any of the following questions are yes, then there should be a more thorough assessment:

- **C = *Control or Cut down*.** Does the patient make attempts to control his or her drinking? Has he or she ever tried to cut down? What was the result? Does the patient ever drink more than intended? Can the patient stop without difficulty after a predetermined number of drinks?
- **A = *Anger*.** If someone suggests to the patient that he or she might be drinking too much, or have a drinking problem, does he or she get angry?
- **G = *Guilt*.** Does the patient feel guilty about the amount he or she drinks?
- **E = *Eye-opener*.** Does the patient need a drink as an eye-opener in the morning, to get going? Does the patient need to drink to feel normal?

Don't forget those scripts! It's easy to concentrate on alcohol and street drugs and forget about addictive prescription drugs. Managed care and employee assistance programs are very concerned about prescription drug abuse, which can create safety hazards and decreased productivity in the workplace. There are many healthcare employees with ready access to pills in the course of their jobs. These "impaired professionals" often have special treatment requirements imposed by their employer and/or state licensing board(s), which will be communicated by the case manager.

Managed care and employee assistance programs are very concerned about prescription drug abuse, which can create safety hazards and decreased productivity in the workplace.

Such prescriptions can also be hazardous to the recovery of clients with a history of substance abuse. If, for example, a client recovering from alcohol dependence is later prescribed Valium or Xanax for anxiety, there is a risk of immediate re-addiction because of the phenomenon of *cross-tolerance*. Current substance abuse (or even any use at all) can also pose risks when clients are prescribed certain types of medication.

Outpatient Individual Therapy?

Several managed care companies' medical necessity guidelines come right out and say that outpatient individual therapy might not be appropriate for substance abuse. Although it sounds as if the managed care company is being directive of treatment, from a clinical perspective it's generally true. Clients in the first year or two of recovery typically need a higher level of structure than is offered by weekly outpatient therapy. They need a group of some kind; if not self-help, then an aftercare or private therapy group. Groups offer clients the chance to connect with others in their situation, to break down the isolation built up during their using careers, and are typically much more effective at combating the frequent denial, minimization, and bargaining of newly sober individuals. Outpatient individual therapy works best when the client has stabilized and has had several months' sobriety; plus, it usually should be in conjunction with any or all of the following: marital/family therapy, 12-step groups, aftercare, or other group. Case managers will question any treatment plan for substance abuse recovery where the only intervention is individual therapy.

Case managers will question any treatment plan for substance abuse recovery where the only intervention is individual therapy.

These clauses in medical necessity codes also should be interpreted to mean that the company is actually reserving the right to suggest a higher level of care. As a case manager, I was frequently in a position to make such a suggestion. Invariably, the response I got was, "Wow, a managed care company that actually cares! I was seeing the client in outpatient because I didn't think you guys would pay for anything else."

What about requesting outpatient therapy for a client who is still using and refuses other treatment? Sometimes clients in denial will ask to try outpatient individual therapy first. Therapists who want to use outpatient therapy to try to break down denial, or who have a client who is still using but refusing a higher level of care, can generally obtain approval. The key, as always, is in the documentation. There are two ideas that must be conveyed:

1. "I have recommended [IOP, Partial, IP] to Bill W., but he refuses to go. He wants to try outpatient and going to AA."
2. "The goal of Bill's outpatient therapy will be to confront his denial that his drinking [and/or using drugs] has had negative consequences in his life, and to help him accept the fact that in order to fix his problems he will never be able to drink [use] again. Will continue to encourage him to accept referral to more specialized substance abuse treatment and AA [NA, CA, etc.]."

These statements convey an understanding of the importance of using different levels and intensities of treatment, depending on the client's circumstances and clinical presentation.

12-Step Groups

If any type of substance abuse is mentioned as a diagnosis or problem, a 12-step group should be listed as an intervention on the treatment plan. If it is not, expect a call or note from the case manager.

What if the client refuses to go? Put it on the treatment plan anyway. Dishonest? Not in the least. If the client refuses, then the subject was obviously brought up during a session. And if it was discussed with the client, then by definition it was part of the treatment plan. The managed care company, despite their performance guarantees, can only attempt to control whether therapists document that they made the recommendation; not whether the client ultimately goes. The written treatment plan indicates what the therapist will recommend for the client (or has already recommended), not what the client ultimately chooses to do or not do. If an assessment is made that a 12-step group is contraindicated, be sure to explain why.

Once a person does have a substance abuse history, there are some managed care types who will forever see them as being in relapse if they don't go to AA or NA daily—even after years and years of clean and sober living. If a client with substantial recovery (5 years or more) has chosen to discontinue participation in 12-step programs, and the presenting problem is not related to substance abuse, his or her recovery, or after-effects from his or her using career, then carefully consider whether a substance abuse in remission diagnosis should be listed at all.

The Controlled Use Controversy

It can be an effective intervention for clients in denial, to predetermine a limit with them and get the client to agree that should he or she be unable to keep to this limit, he or she will seek more specialized substance abuse treatment and/or go to a 12-step group. But for recovering clients, it's a clinical controversy as to whether they can and/or should successfully engage in controlled use as opposed to 100 percent abstinence. While I don't pretend to have the clinical answer, it's probably a good idea for the purposes of managed care not to include any treatment goals that say, "Patient will be able to drink no more than 'x' amount per week," or "Patient to be able to drink/use recreationally." Better safe than sorry, when it comes to obtaining authorization for a client's treatment.

If any type of substance abuse is mentioned as a diagnosis or problem, a 12-step group should be listed as an intervention on the treatment plan. If it is not, expect a call or note from the case manager.

Personality Disorders

*Some benefit
plans actually
state that
personality
disorders are
excluded
conditions.*

Some therapists think that giving an Axis II diagnosis helps the case for medical necessity. Unfortunately, it does not. In fact, some benefit plans actually state that personality disorders are excluded conditions. They typically allow coverage of patients with Axis II diagnoses only if the treatment plan is focused on a concomitant Axis I disorder.

Beware of Diagnosing on Axis II

There's a reason for the suspicion of personality disorders, namely, the belief that characterological difficulties cannot be impacted significantly by short-term, problem-focused psychotherapy, and that effective treatment takes years, a kind of "Woody Allen syndrome." Wherever possible, avoid giving Axis II diagnoses to managed care patients.

Special Exception: Dialectical Behavior Therapy (DBT)

Borderline personality disorder can be very expensive to treat. Just managing these patients safely may require multiple hospitalizations, which are expensive even if the stays are very brief. Typically, borderline patients have one or more Axis I diagnoses for which treatment may be authorized by managed care. However, not reimbursing direct treatment of the personality disorder component seems analogous to authorizing bypass surgery for a heart attack but then refusing to allow the doctor to monitor blood pressure. Because of the acting out inherent in borderline personality, untreated BPD may actually exacerbate Axis I diagnoses such as depression, anxiety, OCD, eating disorders, substance abuse, and so forth. For this reason, managed care companies are often willing to reimburse for Linehan-model dialectical behavior therapy, a cognitive-behavioral group treatment model that has been shown to have good results in helping borderlines maintain their functioning and minimize acting out.

Experimental Procedures and Managed Care

Do the clinical aspects of experimental or "alternative" techniques get a "fair hearing" from managed care? Eye Movement Desensitization and Reprocessing (EMDR) for instance, is still not directly approved by several of the largest carve-out managed behavioral care firms (*Practice*

Strategies, March 1999), which have classified EMDR as an experimental technique. With the total absence of regulation in managed care's first decade, the companies have, so far, been able to protect the process by which they determine the procedures that will be covered, under the guise of "proprietary" information.

Managed behavioral care organizations are now required by NCQA to develop and implement technology assessment guidelines (NCQA, 2000, UM 7). However, NCQA does not require that the internal technology assessment guidelines be made readily available to any consumer or professional who asks to see them. It certainly lends credence to Ivan Miller's (1996) criticism that "the managed care industry is the master of the NCQA *watchdog* [sic], and this dog is guarding the industry's profits from the proponents of true accountability and effective regulation."

NCQA does not require that the internal technology assessment guidelines be made readily available to any consumer or professional who asks to see them.

The answer isn't going to come from NCQA. Instead, as patients begin to win the rights to sue their health plans and ERISA continues to be challenged, managed care will begin to sit up and take notice. In the spring of 1999 Aetna U.S. Healthcare lost a lawsuit, *Goodrich vs. Aetna,* in San Bernardino, California. The patient, David Goodrich, had been denied coverage of cancer treatments, which Aetna claimed were experimental. The jury sided with his widow, and because Mr. Goodrich had been a government employee (thus exempt from ERISA), the jury was able to award punitive damages to Aetna in the amount of $116 million (Grinfeld, 1999).

Psychological Testing

It's not easy to get it approved. Testing is rarely authorized by managed care companies, even in plans with more generous benefits. Most medical necessity guidelines generally say that unless psychological testing can (1) be used to help clarify a diagnosis/disorder, and (2) the results of the testing will aid in treatment planning, it isn't going to be reimbursed. Then it gets worse. Typically, the psychologist doing the testing will be expected to justify why each particular test is needed. The questions asked by the reviewer will go something like this:

Most medical necessity guidelines say that unless psychological testing can (1) be used to help clarify a diagnosis/ disorder, and (2) the results of the testing will aid in treatment planning, it isn't going to be reimbursed.

1. Why are the results from each requested test necessary for aid in developing the treatment plan (or, phrased differently, "How will the results of each test improve the treatment plan?")?

2. What information is likely to be obtained from each requested test that cannot be obtained by a clinical interview, a client self-report scale, a collateral interview, or some other (cheaper) method?

3. Why have all the other methods been inadequate to get the needed information?

4. Why is this information needed to develop the treatment plan?

Projective tests are rarely authorized, and the nonprojective personality tests don't fare a whole lot better.

So what does this mean? Well, for starters, that those Rorschachs and TATs will be collecting dust on the shelf, unless the client will agree to pay out-of-pocket. Projective tests are rarely authorized, and the nonprojective personality tests don't fare a whole lot better. Not necessarily because of the nature of the tests (although the projective method and the theory behind it isn't popular with managed care), but because what the tests are measuring isn't likely to be judged useful in answering any of the above questions.

"Johnny just isn't doing well in school . . . could he maybe have ADHD?" School systems are overburdened with requests for testing: for ADHD, for other behavioral problems, for underachievement, for learning disabilities, for gifted programs. Parents who are concerned about the quality of their children's education, and attempt to circumvent the bureaucracy of the school system, end up facing another bureaucracy known as the managed behavioral healthcare organization. There, they frequently have access only to a master's level case manager with no education, credentials, or experience in psychological testing. Although the actual decisions about requests for testing are made by a staff psychologist, it's not at all uncommon for the master's level case manager to be the one who has to communicate to Johnny's mother why GenRUs Behavioral Healthcare won't pay for him to be tested for ADHD.

Managed care company utilization review guidelines specifically exclude educational testing. It's not just the fault of the managed care companies, though; even if the medical necessity guidelines didn't exclude it, it's a rare benefit plan that would pay for educational testing in this day and age. But the boundaries between educational and mental health are a whole lot fuzzier than they might appear to be at first glance. A request to test 8-year-old Sally who is still struggling with reading, but who has no mental health or attentional symptoms, is fairly obvious; she might be dyslexic, or have a reading disorder of some kind. But what about when a child has educational problems that may be caused by an underlying emotional or behavioral disorder, or even family problems that are contributing to academic underachievement? When the distinction between educational and mental health isn't clear, often the managed care company will make the determination based on how the test results will be used. In the case of ADHD, they might ask, will the tests really help the psychiatric treatment plan, or will they be used to form a basis for school placement or for the development of individualized education plans (IEPs)?

One Exception

Neuropsychological testing is the easiest of all, in terms of obtaining managed care approval, because these tests are much more likely to meet the medical necessity criteria. Which makes sense. If a patient suffered a head injury in a car accident, or is partially paralyzed as a result of a stroke, neuropsych testing can help clarify the extent of the damage to cognitive and motor functions, as well as get an idea of what capabilities the patient still has. Moreover, the victim of an accident or stroke can't always say what is wrong in a clinical interview, as verbal and cognitive functioning may be affected. They require the testing to identify the problems, because there often is no other cheaper way. The results of the tests thus directly impact the treatment (rehabilitation) plan, because the tests are identifying the problems the treatment plan will be aimed at solving.

It probably doesn't hurt that under many insurance plans, neuropsychological testing is paid for by the medical benefits! This can be problematic, though, as well as advantageous, if behavioral health benefits are carved out, because each side may deny the claims stating that the other one is expected to pay, leaving the frustrated patient and his or her family holding the bill.

Attempting to Get Psychological Testing Authorized

First, find out the specific managed care company's policy and procedure(s) regarding requests for testing. Don't ask the client to call. Although it's more hassle to make the call in the short run, in the long run it will save time. Asking a client and/or a family member to undertake calling for information is like asking for a miscommunication to occur, because the client/family member might not understand the case manager's explanation of how medical necessity for testing is determined.

When the distinction between educational and mental health isn't clear, often the managed care company will make the determination based on how the test results will be used.

Allow at least a week to obtain the authorization prior to beginning the testing.

If there are any questions about the request, ask to confer directly with the reviewing psychologist.

Allow at least a week to obtain the authorization prior to beginning the testing. It's completely unfair to the client to schedule the test for a Tuesday and then tell the client or his or her family to call the managed care company on Monday for precertification. This sets everyone up for a bad experience.

After completing any required paperwork, get the name, credentials, and extension of the person who will be reviewing the request. If there are any questions about the request, ask to confer directly with the reviewing psychologist. I think of it as being like the children's game of "Telephone." Too many people relaying messages causes a breakdown in the accuracy of the message when it reaches its intended recipient. If the psychologist employed by the managed care company isn't too busy to review requests, then he or she isn't too busy to speak directly with the requestor as part of that review. Here are a few guidelines:

- Know exactly which tests are going to be needed.
- Know exactly how many billable hours will be needed to cover not just the administration of the test(s), but also scoring, report writing, and explanation of findings to the client/family.
- Build these hours into the request from the very beginning; coming back later for an additional authorization to cover these costs almost never works.
- Expect that the managed care company will ask to see a copy of the full report, and obtain the client/family's permission.
- Managed care companies do not authorize testing that will be used to determine which medications to prescribe, or whether to prescribe medication at all.
- Do not expect a managed care company to pay for testing on an "emergency" basis. As my colleague Neil Horowitz, PhD, who reviews testing requests for Merit Behavioral Care (now part of Magellan), puts it, "No one will die as a result of not being given immediate psych testing."

12

Denials and Appeals

Joe Plocica was a 68-year-old male with a long history of major depression. In the past, he had attempted suicide. . . . In March of 1997, he had overdosed on alcohol and Halcyon, at which time he underwent inpatient care. . . . On June 25, 1998, Joe Plocica was admitted to John Peter Smith Hospital due to an overdose. He was transferred to the psychiatric floor of All Saints Hospital. . . . He remained in the hospital until July 8, 1998. . . . After discharge on July 8, 1998, Joe was taken early in the morning of July 9, 1998, to All Saints emergency room. Some time during the evening of July 8 or early morning of July 9, he left his bedroom, went to the garage, and proceeded to drink a half-gallon of antifreeze in an attempt to kill himself. Joseph Plocica subsequently died from his self-inflicted injuries on July 17, 1998. (excerpts from *Plocica vs. NYLCare* et al., 1998)

Mr. Plocica was a member of a Medicare HMO, which had carved out its behavioral health portion to one of the largest national managed behavioral health organizations, Merit Behavioral Care (now part of Magellan). His family subsequently filed suit, an option in their state, Texas, since September 1997, when Senate Bill 386 was passed, allowing HMOs and other managed care organizations to be sued for denials of care (Grinfeld, 1998). The central issue of the suit is whether Merit Behavioral Care and the psychiatrist employed by them as utilization reviewer, made a treatment decision that Mr. Plocica was ready to be released, overruling the objections of the patient's psychiatrist. Legally, *Plocica vs. NYLCare* is expected to be a landmark case, regardless of the outcome.

For mental health professionals, Mr. Plocica's case demonstrates why understanding the intricacies of managed care denials and appeals protocol may be a life-or-death matter.

Types of Denials

An administrative denial occurs when there is a failure to fulfill one or more requirements of the insurance plan, and the claim ends up being denied.

There are actually two types of denials. An administrative denial occurs when there is a failure to fulfill one or more requirements of the insurance plan, and the claim ends up being denied. We've all encountered these: The therapist is out-of-network, there was a failure to precertify, there was more than one session per day, the OTR was late, the authorization is expired, the service or diagnosis is not covered under the plan, or the maximum benefit has been paid, and so on. Usually, therapists and clients don't find out until the claim comes back denied. For this reason, administrative denials are sometimes referred to as *claims denials*. Administrative reasons to deny treatment are the major money-savers for managed care: the more hoops placed in the path of the therapist and client in order for benefits to cover therapy, the more likely it is that some will choose not to jump through them.

The clinical denials are the denials of care due to a perceived lack of medical necessity.

The *clinical denials* are the denials of care due to a perceived lack of medical necessity. For example, if a client's benefit plan states that the plan will cover only 20 medically necessary sessions per year, it's an administrative denial if all 20 are certified and then the rest are denied. However, if the client is only authorized 15 of those 20, and then there is a denial due to lack of medical necessity, which occurs after a treatment plan is submitted for re-authorization, that's a clinical denial.

Is It a Real Denial?

Case manager Andrew Reviewer called Mary Caring, LCSW, about an outpatient treatment report for Brenda Brown, who had been seen for 15 sessions. Mary was requesting 10 additional visits. Brenda's diagnoses were Adjustment Disorder Mixed Depression/Anxiety and Dysthymia, resulting from her role as primary caretaker for her elderly mother, who had always been critical and disapproving. Andrew called to get clarification from Mary regarding her treatment plan of helping Brenda to develop better self-esteem, detach from mother's criticism, address guilt and anger, and identify other caretaking solutions. During the conversation with Mary, Andrew remarked that being her mother's caretaker is an ongoing situation for Brenda but that her benefits are for brief, solution-focused therapy only. He authorized 7 more sessions but stated, "I doubt weekly psychotherapy is really going to continue to be medically necessary after that."

Mary reported to Brenda at the next session what Andrew said. Furious, Brenda called Andrew and complained about "being denied."

It's very common for a case manager to hint that sessions will be denied at the next review. Andrew might have thought he was being helpful by letting Mary know his thinking. From the perspective of Mary and Brenda, though, it appeared as if Andrew had already concluded that Brenda's clinical presentation after 7 weeks will not meet medical necessity criteria. It may even be true that Andrew put a special "flag" on the case such that if Mary does send a new OTR, it will be pulled for close scrutiny. However, Andrew's statement in this situation is not a denial. For one thing, it's not possible to determine whether Brenda will meet medical necessity criteria seven weeks later. Medical necessity determinations are always based on the clinical picture of the client at the time of the review. Andrew did authorize sessions, and did not communicate, in writing, an intent to deny in the future.

Medical necessity determinations are always based on the clinical picture of the client at the time of the review.

A real denial must be communicated in writing. There are no exceptions. This is a requirement of all the major accreditation organizations, most states, and the Federal Employee Retirement and Income Security Act, better known as ERISA. According to attorney Robert Perez of the Health Administration Responsibility Project (HARP) advocacy organization (1996), the written denial letter must have these characteristics to be compliant with ERISA:

1. It must be in language that is easily understood by the layperson.
2. The specific reason for the denial must be included in the letter.
3. The letter must cite the provision from the Summary Plan Description that applies to the denial.
4. The letter must describe what additional information would have resulted in a payment of the claim.
5. The letter must describe the appeals process.

The burden of denial belongs to the managed care company. Such comments by case managers are not to be considered an official denial of authorization; however, hearing these comments may cause therapists to end up frustrated and conclude that there's no point in going through the utilization review process if it's going to end in a denial. This is a trap—don't fall into it! It doesn't matter what a case manager has said in

Therapists who sign managed care contracts and accept managed care patients, have also accepted the obligation to advocate for coverage for treatment that is necessary in their clinical opinion.

The first thing to understand about a managed care denial is that it is a process, not an event. There are clearly defined steps which the managed care company must take in issuing a denial.

Case managers do not have the authority to issue a denial in any managed behavioral care company.

an earlier review, if the therapist doesn't submit a formal request for re-authorization, the managed care company is saved from having to deny. Therapists who sign managed care contracts and accept managed care patients, have also accepted the obligation to advocate for coverage for treatment that is necessary in their clinical opinion. Failure to do so may constitute malpractice (Bernstein & Hartsell, 1998).

It's not a good idea to share a case manager's comments with the client. It needlessly exacerbates the triangulation inherent to providing therapy in a managed care context. Mary's having told Brenda served no purpose other than for her to get upset.

If the case manager makes such a statement, it's okay to ask him or her directly, "Can you please explain why you think that further therapy will not be medically necessary at the time of the next review?" It might be that by listening to the case manager's reasoning, a denial at the next review can actually be avoided if the case is presented according to the case manager's recommendations.

The Denial Process

The first thing to understand about a managed care denial is that it is a process, not an event. There are clearly defined steps which the managed care company must take in issuing a denial. These procedures do not vary much, if at all, between companies, since they are mandated by a variety of sources: ERISA, state laws, and accreditation organizations such as NCQA, JCAHO, and URAC (Utilization Review Accreditation Commission).

Contrary to popular belief, case managers do not have the authority to issue a denial in any managed behavioral care company. The reason is that most case managers are clinicians with some form of master's degree, and NCQA standards state that "A psychiatrist, doctoral level clinical psychologist, or certified addiction medicine specialist reviews any denial that is based on clinical appropriateness" (NCQA, 2000, UM 3.2). Even where the case manager is a PhD, the company typically is going to make very sure that every denial, even for outpatient treatment, is reviewed by a senior clinical management staff member, in order to decrease the company's liability. A case manager who thinks that an OTR doesn't reflect adequate medical necessity according to the managed care company's standards must pass the case on for further review.

Pending Denial

The process of additional review of the case by a company psychiatrist or psychologist is known as a *pending denial,* meaning that the managed care company is considering denying, but whether or not they actually end up issuing a formal denial depends on what the treating practitioner has to say. If a case manager calls a therapist about an OTR that was submitted and says, "I'd like you to talk with our staff psychiatrist or psychologist about this," this might be a signal that the managed care company is seriously considering denying treatment. There are other reasons a case manager might want a senior clinical adviser to review a case in more detail with a therapist, so if the reason for the additional review is not made clear at the time the case manager requests it, therapists should ask directly, "Is this a pending denial?"

The pending denial period is the amount of time given to the treating clinician to connect with the managed care representative for the additional review, which is known as a *peer-to-peer review.* It is customary that treatment held during the pending denial period will be authorized and reimbursed, so as not to penalize the patient for the delay imposed by the need for additional utilization review.

It is customary that treatment held during the pending denial period will be authorized and reimbursed, so as not to penalize the patient for the delay imposed by the need for additional utilization review.

Denial protocol is largely based on inpatient treatment, which is where most denials occur. It is frequently the case that what is a matter of well-established custom and routine for hospitalizations is fuzzy and vague when it comes to outpatient psychotherapy. For inpatient treatment, the standard pending denial period is 24 hours, or one hospital day. For outpatient treatment, there isn't a standard pending denial time period, which leaves it up to the managed care company, or even the senior clinical advisor, to set the limit.

There's an easy solution that can be adopted. If the unit of service for inpatient treatment is one hospital day, then the unit of service for outpatient is one session. Since the typical frequency of outpatient visits is once weekly, outpatient pending denial periods should last a full five working days, and the managed care company should reimburse for the session held during the week of the pending denial period.

Documenting Denials

It is absolutely imperative to begin documenting everything, from the moment the case manager utters the words *pending denial* or requests a peer review. Who, what happened, when, and how each step in the process unfolded is vital. Appeals have been won on the ability of the therapist and/or client to demonstrate that the managed care company has made critical mistakes. A complete record also serves as evidence that the therapist did everything possible to advocate for the client.

Appeals have been won on the ability of the therapist and/or client to demonstrate that the managed care company has made critical mistakes.

> August 2, 1999, 2:30 P.M. Call from case manager Bea Worker of GenRUs Behavioral Health informing that GBH is issuing pending denial for Jane Jones. GBH concern is that client is ready to be discharged. Ms. Worker requested this therapist have peer review with Eric Adams PhD by close of business August 10, 1999. Dr. Adams at (888) 888-8888 ext. 88.

> August 2, 1999, 2:45 P.M. Left voice mail for Eric Adams PhD requesting to schedule peer review ASAP. Left office & pager numbers for return call.

> August 3, 1999, 10 A.M. Voice mail from Eric Adams, PhD of GBH leaving several times to schedule peer review. Called back, selected time of 11 A.M. on Friday Aug. 6, left voice mail with time selection.

The Peer-to-Peer Review

The managed care company's peer reviewer must have the same or higher credentials than the treating clinician.

Who reviews the case? For everyone except psychiatrists, outpatient peer-to-peer reviews are most likely to be conducted with a psychologist, since the MDs employed by the managed care company are busy with inpatient and other higher levels of care. If the treating clinician is a psychiatrist, though, the review should be with one of the company's psychiatrists, since the managed care company's peer reviewer must have the same or higher credentials than the treating clinician.

Preparing for the Review

Asking what questions the managed care company has is the best way to prepare.

What's the question? Asking what questions the managed care company has is the best way to prepare. When a case manager informs a therapist of a pending denial and requests a peer review, he or she should be able to identify the managed care company's concerns about authorizing continued treatment.

> You've seen Jane Jones for 40 sessions, but there doesn't seem to be much more progress now than there was three months ago, and you're still asking for weekly sessions. She seems to be doing well enough, so that's what we want to discuss.

By getting this information from the case manager ahead of time, the therapist and Jane can meet to discuss whether or not Jane really does continue to need weekly visits, and identify why. What are the goals, and what will Jane accomplish, by meeting weekly instead of less often?

If for some reason the case manager doesn't identify a central question for review, don't hesitate—call the case manager back to ask!

Use the Company's Medical Necessity Guidelines

Refer to the medical necessity guidelines of the particular managed care company. Try to find justification for continued treatment according to these guidelines; this is the document that the reviewers are using (see Chapter 7). Then write it down, with reference to the specific guideline that supports the case. Consider writing down the key points that must be communicated, so as not to forget when actually engaged in the review. Practice with a colleague or supervisor who can offer feedback, or who can play the role of the managed care psychologist/psychiatrist.

During the Review

Listen to the reviewer's questions; they may be originating from mistaken impressions made by the OTR, which he or she will have seen. The peer review is a chance to correct any miscommunications about the patient's status. Focus on concrete, behavioral symptoms and impairments in daily functioning. Avoid concepts such as resolving transference and so forth (see Chapters 9 and 10).

The Negotiation Dilemma

The peer reviewer may try to "cut a deal." Managed care companies like to be able to say in denial letters that although they denied the requested treatment, level, or frequency of care due to lack of medical necessity, they offered an alternate treatment option which they would pay for. Whether or not to negotiate can be tricky. Let's say, for example, that Dr. Smith, the therapist treating Jane Jones, meets with Jane in preparation for the review and Jane becomes tearful and anxious, almost panicky, at the thought of terminating therapy. Dr. Smith and Jane conclude that weekly sessions are still necessary. During the review, though, the company's psychologist offers a compromise: GenRUs

Managed care companies like to be able to say in denial letters that although they denied the requested treatment, level, or frequency of care due to lack of medical necessity, they offered an alternate treatment option which they would pay for.

Behavioral Health will pay for twice-monthly sessions. Should Dr. Smith accept the deal?

The initial instinct would probably be to accept the offer. After all, GBH is indicating that they are willing to pay for twice-monthly visits rather than cutting Jane off completely. That means that at least half of Jane's sessions would be paid. Half is better than nothing, right?

Not from the perspective of Dr. Smith's malpractice liability. Here's why: Dr. Smith and Jane have determined together that Jane needs weekly sessions, and this is what has been documented in her case notes. The negotiation dilemma in peer reviews is that a therapist who accepts less than what has been documented is his or her minimum recommendation for level/frequency of treatment, is abandoning his or her duty to advocate for the client. Suppose Dr. Smith were to find herself on the stand as a defendant in a malpractice action because something happened to Jane. Jane's lawyer asks:

> Dr. Smith, it says here in the record that you believed Jane needed to be seen weekly. So why didn't you appeal the managed care company's decision to authorize twice-monthly sessions?

How is Dr. Smith to answer the lawyer's question?

When therapists accept a managed care company's negotiated offer, the liability rests with the therapist, not with the company, because if the deal is accepted, there is no denial which can then be appealed. Therapists who accept a negotiated deal in a peer review should be very sure that whatever is agreed to conforms with the clinical recommendations for the client which have already been documented in that client's chart. If the managed care company's offer is less than a therapist's documented recommendations, the offer should be politely declined. The reviewer will then proceed with the denial, so that an appeal can be made.

Clients can safely do what therapists cannot. Let's say Dr. Smith cannot convince Dr. Adams to authorize weekly sessions, and so the denial is issued. In the denial letter to Jane and Dr. Smith, Dr. Adams indicates that sessions twice monthly are being offered as an alternative to weekly visits. Suppose Jane decides, after thinking about her options, that she'd rather not go to the trouble of appealing, and she informs Dr. Smith and her case manager of her decision. This gets Dr. Smith off the hook, since Jane is the one who made the decision to accept the managed care company's offer of

The negotiation dilemma in peer reviews is that a therapist who accepts less than what has been documented is his or her minimum recommendation for level/ frequency of treatment, is abandoning his or her duty to advocate for the client.

less treatment than what Dr. Smith recommended. Dr. Smith should, of course, document the sequence of events carefully and thoroughly.

10 Things to Avoid in a Peer-to-Peer Review

1. Threatening a lawsuit.
2. Getting into a credentials-comparison match with the reviewer.
3. Making statements to the effect that "it's all your fault if the client commits suicide/decompensates/relapses." Or, prophesying the suicide/decompensation/relapse of the client if the denial goes through.
4. Taking the "moral high ground" in the conversation due to not being employed by the managed care company.
5. Threatening to resign from the network if the denial goes through.
6. Making any sort of statement about how evil (*heartless, greedy, etc.*) the company is for denying care.
7. Telling the managed care psychologist or psychiatrist that he or can't make a fair determination without evaluating the patient face to face.
8. Threatening to have the patient call their benefit administrator if the denial goes through, threatening to go to the media, to notify prominent politicians, and so on.
9. Audiotaping the conversation for the patient, or doing the review with the patient in the room.
10. Threatening to report the reviewer to his or her state licensing board or professional association.

Unprofessional behavior, often the result of years of understandable anger and frustration with managed care, hurts the client as much as it hurts the practitioner, and doesn't change the managed care system. Keep the tone of the peer review collegial wherever possible.

The Denial Letter

The managed care company must notify both the client and therapist of a denial in writing, and the denial letter must include instructions and timeframes for filing an appeal. Most managed care companies allow only a specific window of time to file an appeal, usually 30 to 60 days. If

The managed care company must notify both the client and therapist of a denial in writing, and the denial letter must include instructions and timeframes for filing an appeal.

there is no response in the form of an appeal, the matter is considered closed and the client will find it almost impossible to get the company to reopen it. For inpatient and other higher levels of care, managed care companies are additionally required to offer expedited appeals due to the clinical urgency of the situation.

Lost in the mail? Not likely. Denial letters are expected to go out to both the therapist and the client within a day of the decision, per NCQA (see Table 12.1). Usually the letters are sent through one of the overnight carriers, although NCQA does allow for electronic notification. Document the arrival (or lack thereof) of the formal denial letter, and ask the client if his or her copy was received, and when.

The Appeals Process

Be sure to document encouraging the client to appeal, and offering to help with the appeal process.

Document educating the client about his or her rights.

The client will need to consent to the appeal, if he or she is capable of giving informed consent. Always get the patient's or parent/guardian's verbal or written permission before initiating an appeal on the patient's behalf.

What if the client refuses to file an appeal? In that case, there's nothing more a practitioner can do. But, be sure to document encouraging the client to appeal, and offering to help with the appeal process (i.e., writing the initial appeal letter together, calling together to initiate the appeal). Document educating the client about his or her rights. For example, Dr. Smith might note:

> August 12, 1999. Session with Jane Jones from 1–2 P.M. Discussed whether to appeal GBH's decision to deny weekly sessions. Jane reluctant to appeal, stating "I'd rather get something than nothing." Explained to Jane that if GBH had authorized 2 sessions per month as "medically necessary," this offer would not be withdrawn just because she appealed. Suggested we call the state Department of Insurance together to ask about state regulations governing managed care denials and appeals. However, Jane decided not to pursue the appeal, but to continue with weekly sessions, paying for every other session out-of-pocket.

Filing the Appeal

Some companies require the patient/family to initiate appeal proceedings; others allow the practitioner to file on behalf of the client. The

Table 12.1
Critical Utilization Review/Appeal Timelines, per NCQA

Precertification:

- The managed care company has 2 working days after receipt of information to authorize/deny precertification of routine cases, and 1 working day to notify the practitioner/member (UM 4.1.1 & UM 4.1.2).
- The managed care company has 1 calendar day (24 hours) to authorize/deny precertification of urgent/emergent cases AND notify the practitioner/facility and member (UM 4.1.4).
- The managed care company must offer an expedited appeal process for urgent situations if there is a denial of coverage, and this must be offered at the time the member/practitioner is notified of the denial (UM 4.1.5).

Concurrent Review (requests for continuing treatment):

- [Inpatient, residential, and intensive outpatient treatment] The managed care company has 1 working day to decide to authorize/deny continued services once the clinical information for the review is received, and 1 working day to notify (UM 4.1.7.1 & UM 4.1.8).
- [Outpatient] The managed care company has 10 working days to make a decision once all necessary information (i.e., OTRs) is received, and 1 working day to notify (UM 4.1.7.2 & UM 4.1.8).
- Managed care companies must offer an expedited appeal for any denial of continuing treatment (UM 4.1.10).

Appeals:

- "Expedited Appeal" means that a decision will be made on the appeal and communicated to the member/practitioner/facility within 72 hours. Decisions communicated orally during this period must be followed up in writing within 2 working days (UM 4.2.2 & UM 4.2.3).
- Standard first-level appeals must be decided within 30 days (note: there is a 15 day grace period to allow for circumstances beyond the company's control) and must be reviewed by a clinician not involved in the original denial (RR 3.2.4.1 & 3.2.4.2).
- If a plan offers a second-level appeal, the second-level appeal must be reviewed by a panel of clinicians not involved in either the original denial or the first-level appeal (RR 3.3.3.1).
- Standard second-level appeals must be reviewed within 30 days and a decision communicated in writing no more than 5 working days following the review (RR 3.3.3.3 & RR 3.3.4).
- Members have the right to appear in person for the second-level appeal hearing (or the first, if no second-level is offered by the plan) or be given the opportunity to communicate directly with the appeal panel by conference call (RR 3.3.3.2 & RR 3.3.3.4).

Note: Length of "pending denial" periods is not specified by the NCQA.

Adapted from NCQA (2000) *Standards and Surveyor Guidelines for the Accreditation of MBHOs.* © NCQA. Used with permission. Numbers following the entries correspond to the section and standard number for easy reference within the document.

If the client is willing and able, it's a good idea for the client to write a letter as well, explaining in his or her own words why continuing in treatment is necessary.

If the client becomes depressed, anxious, or otherwise impaired due to the denial and/or the stress of the appeals process, the therapist should communicate this at once to the managed care company.

logistical details of appeal procedure may vary somewhat depending on the specific managed care company. For example, one company may allow the practitioner or patient to start an appeal simply by calling the appeals department, whereas another may require receipt of a request for an appeal in writing.

Once the appeal is filed, the therapist and client will be asked to submit whatever additional records, written testimonials, evidence, and so on that supports their case. Sometimes there is a form for the therapist to complete, but it is more usual for a therapist to write a letter. At the first appeal, some managed care companies will request the client's entire file, including case notes; others won't require the full chart until a later level of appeal, or at all. If the client is willing and able, it's a good idea for the client to write a letter as well, explaining in his or her own words why continuing in treatment is necessary. Collateral written statements indicating the need for continuing treatment from one or more family members and/or the patient's primary care physician, might also lend weight.

If the client becomes depressed, anxious, or otherwise impaired due to the denial and/or the stress of the appeals process, the therapist should communicate this at once to the managed care company, and this information will play a role in whether or not the original denial is overturned.

Continue to document the course of the appeal by indicating the dates materials were received and each and every communication with representatives of the managed care company about the case. Always be sure to include name of the employee, position/credentials, phone number with extension, time/date, and nature of the interaction, in the client's file.

Point out procedural errors. If the denial letters didn't arrive on time, or if there was some other obvious error made by the company in either the denial or the utilization review process, it's certainly worth letting someone in the appeals department know as part of the first level of appeal. Don't wait until the clinical appeal is settled before introducing grievances about the company's handling of the case: it may help bolster the client's chances of getting the denial overturned, or at least getting some additional payment made due to procedural error(s) by the managed care company.

If procedural problems with regard to the way the company has handled any part of the case become part of an appeal, be sure to state an opinion as to how the managed care company might fairly redress the grievance, even if the denial is upheld. Managed care companies are required to track and resolve complaints about their performance, but they won't know what the client and/or practitioner thinks is a fair solution unless one is suggested.

John Doe was sent by his company to be an on-site consultant at a plant about five hundred miles away. The assignment was to last at least a year. John struggled with loneliness and depression after the transfer. The year before, John had been in therapy with Bill Holmes, LCSW, a therapist on his managed care company's network. John called the company, wanting authorization to resume sessions with Bill, by phone. Their first appointment was scheduled for that same evening. The intake clinician did not know whether such a special situation would be covered, and offered to send John a list of network therapists in his new location. John refused, and the intake clinician transferred John to the case manager assigned to John's state.

John left the case manager a detailed voice mail, which, because of work overload, she did not hear until two days later. There was then a delay in the case manager getting to consult with her supervisor. Three more days later, the supervisor determined that ongoing telephone sessions were not appropriate and that John should instead either use the EAP or find a therapist in the new city. A full working week had gone by before the managed care company made a decision, and John had already had two telephone sessions. A denial letter was duly sent out and John appealed.

Bill sent a letter with clinical rationale for the phone sessions including a plan for face-to-face medical monitoring of John by his new PCP. John also wrote a letter explaining why continuing to work with Bill would be more beneficial than seeing a new therapist face-to-face. In his letter, John detailed the managed care company's delay in responding to his request. He included facts such as the time and date of his original call, the names of the intake clinician and case manager, and the time and date the case manager finally returned his call. John argued that if the denial was upheld he should be authorized for the first two sessions, because of the delay in precertification, and two more sessions to account for those sessions held during the appeal period.

The psychologist chosen reviewing the appeal decided that phone sessions could not be substituted for face-to-face. However, the appeals director authorized the four phone sessions with Bill due to the delay in precertification and to cover the sessions held during the appeal process.

John's appeal, although not successful in convincing the managed care company to pay for telephone sessions, was well argued on procedural grounds. John, realizing that a managed care company should not have

Don't wait until the clinical appeal is settled before introducing grievances about the company's handling of the case: it may help bolster the client's chances of getting the denial overturned, or at least getting some additional payment made due to procedural error(s) by the managed care company.

*Appeal
departments do
not always get
informed with
regard to the
sequence of events
in the Clinical
and/or Customer
Service
departments.*

an unlimited amount of time to decide on a simple precertification, in-formed the appeals department, as part of the appeal, about the way his case had fallen through the cracks. Appeal departments do not necessar-ily always get informed with regard to the sequence of events in the Clin-ical and/or Customer Service departments. Table 12.1 outlines some of the critical time deadlines in the precertification, utilization review, de-nial, and appeals process, as defined by NCQA.

Jurisdiction

By virtue of needing to remain objective, appeals departments are some-what set apart from life on the front lines in the managed care company. Once a case is formally denied, it passes from the purview of case man-agement and customer service, into the hands of the appeals department. Always work directly with appeals staff after a denial has been made, un-less specifically directed otherwise.

*Always work
directly with
appeals staff after
a denial has been
made, unless
specifically
directed
otherwise.*

If a complaint is made as part of an appeal, the appeals staff is required to investigate the complaint. The complaint, as in John's case, may not in-fluence the clinical decision made in the appeal, but the appeals staff has the authority to resolve the complaint, even if it means partially over-riding an upheld clinical denial based on administrative grounds. If the managed care company is made aware of a crucial error in procedure, it's to their advantage to make amends. They aren't going to want the "bad press" which will result if the consumer goes to his or her employer, state authorities, and/or accreditation organizations with documented reports of mishandled utilization review or precertification decisions.

Who reviews the appeal? The appeals department staff should be willing and able to answer these questions about the appeal reviewer(s):

1. Credentials and expertise.
2. Title and duties of each reviewer's position within the company.
3. If the reviewer(s) are not employed by the managed care company, what is the financial relationship between the reviewer(s) and the managed care company?

For a first-level appeal, the professional who reviews the case is almost always a psychiatrist employed in another area of the managed care company. He or she should not have been involved in the original denial decision in any way, and should know nothing about the case until being brought in to review the appeal.

Many plans offer a second level of appeal. In other words, if the denial is upheld the first time it is appealed, the opportunity is there to get yet another clinical opinion as to the medical necessity of the recommended treatment. Some companies and/or benefit plans even offer a third level of appeal. Make sure to ask how many levels of appeal the client is entitled to.

The Last Chance

At the final level of appeal, the behavioral health professional reviewing the case should not be employed by the managed care company, for obvious reasons. Who knows whether there is a financial incentive to uphold a denial, or pressure to decide in favor of the managed care company out of fear of negative consequences to one's job? But a non-employee may not be as independent as it might seem on the surface, either. Be assertive about inquiring as to the nature of the financial arrangements between an independent reviewing professional and the managed care company. Specifically:

1. Is the professional doing the review also a participating provider on the managed care company's panel? A yes answer means an economic link is present; managed care companies can always stop making referrals if they don't like a verdict on an appeal review.
2. Who pays the reviewer(s)? To the extent that the managed care company is paying, one wonders how "independent" a non-employee professional reviewer can be. It's an inherent conflict of interest to overturn too many denials, or the managed care company will simply choose someone else next time.

The last level of review all depends on the benefit plan. Some benefit purchasers solve the problem of economic independence from the managed care company at the final appeal level by directly retaining one or more clinicians to serve as reviewer(s), thus removing the final appeal from the purview of the managed care company. Or, the employer/union, insurance carrier, or state Medicaid authority will use a consulting firm that employs clinicians. Such consulting firms advise on issues of benefit plan design, and contract to provide professionals for any final-level appeals. Or, the Summary Plan Description (the document describing

Make sure to ask how many levels of appeal the client is entitled to.

At the final level of appeal, the behavioral health professional reviewing the case should not be employed by the managed care company.

the benefit plan in detail) may specify the creation of an appeal review panel staffed by nominations from both the managed care company and the employer/consulting firm, such that any bias in terms of who is paying is canceled out. By the terms of the benefit contract, the managed care company is bound to adhere to whatever decision is reached at the final level of appeal, however that final level is structured.

Some states are enacting legislation mandating the use of independent review panels. Even in states with such laws, though, not all clients may be covered. The state insurance department will be able to determine whether a state's independent-review law covers a particular client. If the insurance plan is underwritten in another state which does not have an independent-review law, or if the client is participating in a self-insured (ERISA) plan, the state DOI, unfortunately, might not have jurisdiction to offer the independent final appeal. (Appendix A lists the contact information for state insurance departments.)

Following the general trend, NCQA's year 2000 accreditation standards (RR 3.6) mandate that MBHO's have an Independent Review program for final-level appeals in place by July 1, 2001. NCQAs specifications indicate that the MBHO should bear the cost of the Independent Review program, and must use an Independent Review Organization (IRO) that is NCQA-certified, unless applicable state law mandates the use of a specific IRO that is not NCQA-accredited.

Beyond the Final Appeal

There is always the option of consulting with an attorney, or the state's department of insurance, at any time during the denial/appeal process.

Many clients may not want to keep fighting; it is energy-draining and prevents them from moving on. It is always the client's choice whether or not to continue through the appeals process and beyond. There is always the option of consulting with an attorney, or the state's department of insurance, at any time during the denial/appeal process. However, the right to sue a health plan is not universal, and it is due to a complicated law known as ERISA.

ERISA

The federal Employee Retirement Income Security Act (ERISA), was passed by Congress in 1974, well before the advent of managed care, and is the dominant law in health care. ERISA applies only to employee benefit plans that are considered self-funded. The quick-and-dirty rule of thumb is that if the employer purchases a prepackaged, commercially available plan from an insurance company or HMO, one that self-employed or uninsured individuals could buy for themselves, then the plan is not self-funded. Instead, it is called *fully-insured*, and the legal jurisdiction is the state's Department of Insurance. *Self-funded* means that the employer has a pool of money set aside to pay for a plan which may be specially designed by the insurer for that particular employer.

ERISA applies only to employee benefit plans that are considered self-funded.

The major ERISA problem is the following: In what is known as the ERISA preemption clause, the states have no jurisdiction for employees covered by self-funded plans. Instead, ERISA beneficiaries should contact the U.S. Department of Labor (see Appendix). However, the federal level typically does not offer the same consumer protections that are available through state Insurance Departments. In terms of lawsuits against health plans, ERISA does not permit damages to be awarded as a result of denial of claims. One can only sue under ERISA to obtain the coverage for the claim (Perez, 1996). Given the high cost of litigation, ERISA thus virtually ensures that no one will take their insurance company to court over a denial of claims.

Disclaimer: There are all kinds of ERISA exceptions and loopholes. The brief description of self-funded versus fully-insured plans given here is for the sole purpose of introducing potential options after appeal levels have been exhausted. It is not meant as a "do-it-yourself" guide to figuring out jurisdiction over a client's benefit plan. Consult an attorney or the state Insurance Department for this purpose. Another good resource is the advocacy group known as HARP (Health Administration Responsibility Project). HARP is a multi-disciplinary group of legal and medical professionals working to enact change to ERISA (see Appendix A for contact information).

Legal challenges are continually being thrown at ERISA, such as the idea that if it can be proved that a managed care organization is actually engaged in the practice of medicine when making utilization review determinations, the managed care organization, like an individual physician, can be sued for malpractice. Additionally, attempts have been made at amending ERISA in Congress. The next few years promise continued developments in the area of managed care liability for utilization review determinations and denials.

13

Getting Paid

Verifying Benefits

The first step to getting paid actually occurs before a claim is submitted, sometimes before a client has ever been to the office. The process of calling to inquire about benefits, eligibility, copayments, limits, and so forth is known as benefits verification, and it would be hard to overstate the importance of this phone call.

The following benefits verification checklist provides a summary of the information that needs to be obtained:

1. Is the patient eligible?
2. What are the mental health/substance abuse benefits?
3. What is the copayment or coinsurance?
4. Is there a deductible? If yes, what is the dollar amount and how much has been used to date?
5. What is the yearly and/or lifetime maximum benefit? How is the maximum expressed: A dollar amount or a session limit? How much/how many have been used to date? If the maximum is yearly, is this a calendar year or based on the anniversary of the first paid claim?
6. Do these benefits apply to any MH/SA professional, or just those in a network? Is the therapist a member of the network? If any MH/SA professional is the answer, be sure to check that the therapist's license type is covered by the plan. Not all licenses are. (Note: Insurance plans generally consider licensure rather than academic degree.)
7. If the therapist is out-of-network, ask for a description of the out-of-network benefits.

8. What is the precertification requirement? Can the therapist take care of it, or is the client required to make the call? Can it be done during this phone call?

9. Is there any concurrent utilization review for medical necessity? If yes, get the details of what will be needed (i.e., written OTRs, phone reviews).

10. If preauthorizing, get the authorization number, if there is one. It will be needed for the claim.

11. Where should claims be sent?

Make a note of the name of the person who verifies the benefits, and the date and keep it in the client's file. Any one of these items could lead to a claims denial. Although at first glance it may seem like a lot, it's quicker and cheaper to do it right the first time than to clean up after billing for months of sessions that may never be paid.

Verification of benefits is not a guarantee of payment. The automated phone menu will play this disclaimer prior to reaching the customer service rep who verifies the benefits. It means exactly what it says: just because the company is giving out benefit information, doesn't mean there's any guarantee the claims will be paid. Whether or not claims are paid is dependent on the patient's eligibility at the time of service and fulfillment of all other administrative requirements (precertification, "participating" network status, etc.). Therapists should be aware that the same disclaimer applies to authorization of sessions. Look at an authorization letter sometime; it's in the fine print.

Just because the company is giving out benefit information, doesn't mean there's any guarantee the claims will be paid.

Eligibility

Eligibility means that the insurance plan is active and all required premiums have been paid. Without eligibility there can be no claims paid. If there is no problem, it can be verified by the customer service rep by a two-second look at the computer. However, under certain circumstances, eligibility might be in some question and cannot be verified during the initial benefits verification call. Or, these same circumstances might result in discontinued eligibility (and thus denied claims) during an authorization period, even if the patient was eligible at the time of the benefits verification call and/or at the time the authorization was issued. For example:

Eligibility means that the insurance plan is active and all required premiums have been paid.

- *Client doesn't pay his or her premium.* Doesn't pay on time or there are complications with the payment process such as a bounced or lost check.
- *COBRA.* COBRA premiums are paid monthly, generally to a benefits organization hired by the employer and unrelated to the MBHO. The entity in charge of the COBRA benefit must then notify the medical plan and/or the managed behavioral carve-out of continued eligibility. Even in the computer age, there is sometimes a delay of a day or so between the time a payment is made for continued COBRA benefits and the time the resulting continued eligibility shows up in the managed care company's computer. Benefit verification calls made during this interval might be unable to determine eligibility.
- *Young adults.* Between the ages of 18 and 25, insurance can be problematic if the patient is covered under a parent's policy. Different health plans have different eligibility rules regarding coverage of young adults. Some require proof of full-time student status; other plans cut off young adults when they reach a certain age, regardless of student status. If a new patient is in this age range and using insurance benefits under a parent's policy, always ask the insurance company what the rules are regarding continued coverage. Young adults can of course obtain COBRA coverage, but there might be gaps in eligibility which result in denied claims for one or more sessions.
- *New calendar year, new insurance.* Don't ever assume a client has the same benefit plan as last year. Companies change benefit packages, and/or people choose different plans during open enrollment. Clients may forget about having opted for new benefits until January's claims come back denied.

> **Getting Paid Survival Tip:** Remember to ask each client at the beginning of a calendar year if he or she has the same insurance plan. If applicable, get a copy of her or his new insurance card, and call to verify benefits.
>
> Even if the client retains the same plan, sometimes features of the plan change. It's safest to reverify at the beginning of each calendar year even if there does not appear to have been any change.

It's a good idea to include a clause in an intake form specifying that if insurance benefits are denied due to terminated eligibility, the patient is responsible for the amount which would have been covered by the insurance or managed care company.

The Vocabulary of Claims

Usual and Customary

Also sometimes referred to as *reasonable and customary* or *usual, customary, and reasonable* charges. It's an important concept. Usual and customary refers to the maximum fee that the insurance company is willing to pay a particular type of professional in a particular region for a particular service. Therapists can, at least in theory, charge anything they want; however, insurance companies aren't going to pay 80 percent of a $300 per hour fee.

Usual and customary fees are determined by an organization called HIAA (Health Insurance Association of America), and are based on studies of actual paid claims. From this data, HIAA determines normative fee ranges per procedure code, per professional license, per geographic area. Managed care companies then buy this data to determine the contract fees they will offer their participating providers.

Usual and customary refers to the maximum fee that the insurance company is willing to pay a particular type of professional in a particular region for a particular service.

All Very Hush-Hush

Insurance companies will never tell professionals or their office staff the amounts that they have determined are usual and customary for that practitioner's license level and geographic area. They do this to protect themselves against the possibility that professionals will fraudulently inflate the bills for their services. If a therapist who normally charges $80 per session finds out that the maximum usual and customary fee for an individual session for that therapist's license is $100, the therapist could potentially bill $100 to get more money, and the insurance company would end up paying more.

Insurance companies will never tell professionals or their office staff the amounts that they have determined are usual and customary for that practitioner's license level and geographic area.

Deductibles

If there is a deductible, it must be met before benefits are paid. Getting information on deductibles for mental health benefits can occasionally involve more than one phone call, if the mental health benefits are carved out but the deductible for mental health is part of the overall medical plan deductible.

Because companies won't release usual and customary figures, knowing how much per session will be contributed to the deductible always takes some guesswork until the explanation of benefits form for the first claim is received. The deductible will be figured at either the usual and customary rate, or the therapist's billed charge (if it should happen to be lower than the maximum usual and customary rate). Or, if the therapist is a contracted member of the network, the session charges contributing to the deductible will be assessed at the therapist's contracted rate.

Copayment versus Coinsurance

They're not exactly interchangeable, although both refer to the portion of the bill paid by the client. Copayments are easier, since there's no waiting for the first paid claim to come back in order to be sure of the exact amount the client owes per session.

Copayment refers to the situation when the patient is required by the insurance plan to pay a certain fixed amount per visit, while co-insurance is when the patient's portion is not fixed, but is a percentage of the bill; for example, 20 percent of charges for services based on usual and customary limitations.

Benefit Years: Redefining the Calendar

A "benefit year" calculates the session limits beginning on the date of service of the first paid claim.

While most health plans still use the calendar year of January 1 to December 31, there are a few that don't. A "benefit year" calculates the session limits beginning on the date of service of the first paid claim.

> Harry and Louise Johnson began marital therapy with Walt Skinner, PhD, in November. Their GenRUs Healthcare Healthy Options HMO benefit book said they were entitled to 20 sessions per year. Harry and Louise figured that they could use 7 or 8 sessions this year and 20 the next, and that should take care of their problems.

Harry and Louise are in for a big shock. In addition to the fact that (1) marital therapy usually isn't covered, and (2) just because a plan brochure advertises 20 sessions per year doesn't mean that all 20 will be authorized as medically necessary, their per year is really a benefit year, not a calendar year. If their first session was November 5, they have 20 sessions as medically necessary to use from November 5 of this year until November 4 of next year. Benefit years are a sneaky way of limiting already-limited benefits just a bit more.

The Mechanics of Billing: Tips for Completing Claim Forms

Use the right form. Although some managed care and insurance companies have designed their own claim forms, the standard form for outpatient services (medical as well as mental health) is the HCFA-1500. It's extremely rare that any insurance or managed care company would reject submission of claims on a HCFA-1500, instead directing that their own form be used. (This does not include EAPs.)

Although some managed care and insurance companies have designed their own claim forms, the standard form for outpatient services (medical as well as mental health) is the HCFA-1500.

HCFA-1500 forms are available from most insurance carriers, medical or general business office supply stores or catalogs, printers, or can be downloaded from the HCFA web site (see Appendix A). Many insurance companies and Medicare carriers now use optical character recognition (OCR) scanning technology. Instead of human data entry, the HCFA-1500 is fed into the computer system, which "reads" the information using the OCR technology, sending the output to the claims examiner. Why is this important? Insurance companies and Medicare carriers using OCR technology require that the HCFA forms be preprinted in a special red ink; otherwise the computer cannot "read" the forms. If this is the case, photocopies, faxed claims, and/or forms printed on a standard laser or ink jet printer will be returned.

Diagnosis code(s) are listed in Box 21 of the HCFA-1500. Technically, Health Care Financing Administration standards require use of the ICD-9-CM, not the *DSM-IV*. ICD-9-CM stands for International Classification of Diseases, Ninth Revision, Clinical Modification, and ICD-9-CM coding materials are available from the American Medical Association. Never heard of it? Don't worry; a copy of the ICD-9-CM isn't generally needed unless the therapist is using an older edition of the *DSM*. Codes in some editions of the *DSM-IV* are actually ICD-9-CM codes: make sure that when purchasing a copy of the *DSM*, the cover bears the notation, "includes ICD-9-CM codes."

Procedure Codes

The procedure codes that are most often used in the mental health field are called the Current Procedural Terminology (CPT) codes, also published by the American Medical Association. Procedure codes and modifiers are listed in Box 24-D of the HCFA-1500 form. Compared to medical procedures, there are actually very few codes for outpatient psychiatry/psychotherapy. Many therapists, particularly those who do no inpatient work or psych testing, make do with the brief description of the common CPT codes often found in managed care company Provider Manuals, and which are always found on contracted fee schedules. However, the CPT coding manual can be a useful reference for practitioners who offer a variety of services.

Accepting Assignment

Managed care contracts expect the therapist to take only a copayment, co-insurance, or deductible from the patient and the rest of the money from the company (known as an exclusive compensation clause).

Accepting assignment (or accepting assignment of benefits) is a technical billing term, meaning that the professional accepts to be paid by the insurance company rather than by the patient. Many therapists, for obvious reasons, prefer that the patient be the one to pay the bill, and then simply file the claims as a service to the patient, expecting the insurance company to reimburse him or her. That's not allowed by managed care contracts, which expect the therapist to take only a copayment, co-insurance, or deductible from the patient and the rest of the money from the company (known as an exclusive compensation clause). Therapists indicate accepting assignment on the HCFA form by checking yes in Box 27 and by having the client sign the consent to assignment of benefits (Box 13; the notation "signature on file" is okay to use if the client has signed a similar statement on the therapist's intake form).

Include the Authorization Number

If the managed care company issues authorization numbers, these generally go in Box 23, and it's a good idea to include them. While one would think that the claims examiner would check the computer system for the presence/absence of an authorization, sometimes they don't. Another alternative is to attach a copy of the authorization letter to the claim.

Contracted or Full Fee?

This is a common question among therapists who have participating-provider contracts with managed care companies. The fee, which goes in Box 24F of the HCFA-1500, technically can either be the contracted rate or the practitioner's full fee. There's no wrong way to do it, although it's advisable to be consistent about which method is being used.

In online queries of several mental health billing experts, most recommended that therapists who have agreed to contracted rates with managed care networks use their full fee on claims. Linda Walker of 1-2-3 Medical Billing in New Jersey, says "Using the full fees also allows the provider to look at the big picture as to what they are losing and allows us to evaluate managed care plans." There is one drawback, though, to using the full fee instead of the contracted. Nancie Lee Cummins, of Medical Management Billing in northern California, states, "Using the larger fee will over inflate your receivables" (i.e., looks as if more money is owed to the therapist than is really the case). For practices that must carefully calculate and adhere to budgets, this might be an important consideration.

Choosing a Billing Method

There are really only four choices:

1. Do the billing by hand.
2. Don't bill—hand the client a superbill and insist on payment in full from the client (not an option for managed care clients).
3. Do the billing using a computer and one of the many software packages commercially available for this purpose.
4. Hire a billing service.

The Superbill Option

Therapists with no managed care contracts can decide not to accept assignment, instead taking the payment from the client. The client then gets a receipt, a *superbill*, and takes care of filing for insurance reimbursement. A superbill is a statement specifically written for clients to file with an insurance company. It includes the therapist's name, address, tax ID, diagnosis, procedure code, and charges, generally has all the codes and fees preprinted, and is a carbon duplicate or triplicate tear-off form. Since the patient is given the superbill to submit to the insurance company, it is an effective method for the therapist to make absolutely sure the patient knows what diagnosis is being submitted, and consents to its release.

For everyone else, the most important consideration is how much time billing takes, and amount of time is related to the proportion of managed care/insurance clients on a caseload. Billing and claims filing tasks are like laundry; they are never completed for long before they need to be done again. Consider not only the time for billing plus actual session hours, but also time needed for other practice-related chores: paperwork, collateral contacts, professional consultation, supervision, phone calls, and (most important of all) marketing. Also, there's always the need to call about denied or delayed claims, no matter how perfectly the forms were completed. Therapists who find themselves procrastinating should consider hiring a billing service, because the first rule of billing is that the longer one waits to bill, the less the chance of ever seeing the payment.

The first rule of billing is that the longer one waits to bill, the less the chance of ever seeing the payment.

Many managed care contracts now set tight turnaround times for therapists to bill, most commonly 60, 90, or 120 days after the session.

Claim Filing Deadlines

Many managed care contracts now set tight turnaround times for therapists to bill, most commonly 60, 90, or 120 days after the session. Timely filing requirements are another reason why therapists who cannot devote enough time to their billing needs, or who tend to procrastinate, should hire a billing service. When claims are denied due to lack of timely filing, therapists are needlessly working for free.

Intro to Electronic Billing: What Therapists Should Know about E-Billing before Deciding Whether to "Do-It-Yourself"

The essence of electronic billing is that the therapist uses billing software and the modem on his or her computer to transmit the claim to a clearinghouse, which modifies the claim to the electronic specifications of the particular insurance/managed care company and transmit it to them.

Electronic claims are much faster, all other things being equal. Depending on the insurance carrier, claims turnaround can be as little as 8 to 14 days with electronically-filed claims, instead of the 30 to 45+ days for paper claims. Here's the catch: the software package chosen by the therapist often limits the choice of clearinghouses.

Does the clearinghouse matter? Yes, not all insurance/managed care companies accept transmissions from all clearinghouses, and not all clearinghouses will transmit to all insurers/managed care companies. Jean Thoensen, of PsychBiller, LLC, in Virginia, specializes in mental health billing. She explains, "What often limits which carriers a clearinghouse will transmit to is claim volume. Are there enough providers willing to submit enough claims to make it worth the clearinghouse's time and money to set up the connection? I've worked with clearinghouses that didn't submit to all Blues because they didn't have enough volume to justify the expense."

Another problem for potential electronic billers, though, is that clearinghouses and software packages which seem solid one year may be gone the next, leaving therapists with an expensive software program that may be unsupported by other clearinghouses, and good only for printing paper claims. Two major companies, InStream and PsychAccess, closed within months of each other in late 1998/early 1999, affecting thousands of therapists (*Practice Strategies*, January 1999).

Not all insurance/managed care companies accept transmissions from all clearinghouses, and not all clearinghouses will transmit to all insurers/managed care companies.

Getting Started

Thoensen advises that practitioners interested in doing their own electronic billing should first be comfortable using the billing program and understand how to use their modem, either to dial up America Online or their Internet Service Provider. The rest, she says, is weighing specific options for cost and convenience and determining which programs/clearinghouses are accepted by the majority of the insurance/managed care companies billed. Thoensen advises calling the insurance companies most regularly billed. The department handling electronic claims will be able to furnish a list of clearinghouses from which they accept transmissions.

Jean Thoensen estimates the costs involved as follows:

- Billing software (minimally about $300 for single user, on up).
- Monthly Internet connection ($15–$25 per month).
- Clearinghouse charges:
  Setup fees (Thoensen says that in her experience these have ranged from $50–$300).
  Per-claim fee (between 25 and 50 cents per claim).

Thoenson advises that clearinghouses "almost always have monthly minimum per-claims charges." Her estimate is that the minimums usually are in the ballpark of 40 to 50 electronic claims per month. It may or may not be cheaper than a stamp.

Some carriers, particularly the government programs and the Blue Cross/Blue Shield companies, offer their own software free or at highly discounted rates to users. Thoensen explains the major advantage and disadvantage of such software: "the claims themselves are free. The advantage of a carrier program is that the claims are sent directly to the carrier's computer system—no middleman. The downside is that you have to enter data in both the billing program and the carrier program."

Bottom line: E-billing may or may not be the most cost-effective method, depending on practice patterns and volume.

Finding the Right Billing Service

It can be an enormous relief to let someone else take over the burden of billing and claims filing, but it can be hard to know who to trust with this most crucial of jobs. The mental health billing experts offered good advice:

- Does this person have any experience with billing and/or the insurance industry? "Too often," says Michelle Alswager of Capitol City Billing and Consulting Services, "this person read an ad in the paper and thought they would give at-home billing a try. I'm not knocking at-home billing . . . I've been doing it for years . . . but there are a lot of start-up'ers out there right now with absolutely no experience." Jean Thoensen, of PsychBiller, LLC, suggests that the biller should attend seminars and training sessions offered by Blue Cross/Blue Shield and governmental carriers.

- Is the at-home biller going to be available? Jean Thoensen says, "A billing service shouldn't be someone who works a full-time day job elsewhere . . . The service has to be available at least a few hours a week to make insurance verification and follow-up telephone calls during business hours."

- Does the biller's business have a dedicated telephone line?

- Does the business project a professional image? This person represents you, and bills under your tax ID. Thoensen suggests asking to see a sample of the statements the biller sends to patients.

- Is electronic billing available?

- Does the billing service have the resources to take on additional clients? Are they expanding too quickly? An impressive array of clients is all very well, but will they have time for you?

- What about confidentiality? Are records kept locked? Who else has access to the computer? Consider using some of the same standards that managed care companies might use on a site visit.

- Does the biller understand how to bill for your services and for the setting in which these services are provided? This is important. Inpatient services are billed under different codes, and often on different forms, than those which are held as an outpatient in the therapist's office.

- If it's a medical billing service, do they understand the special needs of mental health?

- Is practice management consultation available? "Can the billing service suggest improvements in forms, processes, or procedures that would make the therapist's life easier?" asks Jean Thoensen.

- All of the billing experts suggested talking with references.

The Mechanics of Claims Processing (Why Do Claims Get Messed Up?)

Murphy's Law of "anything that can go wrong, will" often seems to be operative. Consider:

- The claims examiner makes a typographical error on a CPT code, professional's billing code/tax ID, date, amount billed, client social security number (or the electronic scanner misreads the data).

- The therapist has multiple billing addresses and the claims processor forgets to look for the address in the system that matches the address where the service was provided.

- Clinical and/or customer service is late in entering an authorization; the claim is received before the authorization is entered into the system so it appears as if there is no authorization (also frequently a problem when claims are paid by a separate company than that which handles the utilization review).

- The claims processor pays according to the wrong benefit plan.

- The employer or COBRA administrator may be late in sending enrollment data to the insurance company, which results in a denial due to lack of eligibility.
- The CPT code used by the therapist doesn't match the one authorized.
- The claims examiner checks the wrong network database and erroneously concludes that the therapist is out-of-network.
- The number of sessions already paid out on an authorization is miscounted.
- The claims processor inadvertently concludes that the patient has reached his or her benefit maximum.
- Charges are incorrectly applied to a deductible that has already been met.
- The claims department's system of interpreting authorization start and end dates differs from the case management department's.
- The claims are repriced and then sent to another company for processing and payment; there are mistakes made in the repricing and/or processing.

An end date is an end date, isn't it? Occasionally, the giving of end dates can result in confusion. If the claims department doesn't communicate with the case managers, then there might be unintended consequences, and it's the therapists who are caught in the crossfire.

Justa Therapist, PhD, was denied payment by UCBH for her client Lolita Nabokov. UCBH had issued these two certifications:

1. 8 sessions, 7/15/98 to 10/15/98.

2. 6 sessions, 10/15/98 to 1/15/99.

Dr. Therapist's ninth session with Lolita was on 10/12/98. Since it was before the beginning date of the second authorization, claims denied it. However, when Dr. Therapist called, she was told that as long as there were no periods of noncertification, claims would simply pay the first 14 visits within the overall date span of 7/15/98 to 1/15/99.

Dr. Therapist appears to be stuck between two departments that haven't agreed on the system to use. Or, it's possible that in theory the two UCBH departments agreed on a policy, but that the individual claims examiner was uninformed, inadequately trained, or simply misunderstood. These sorts of errors happen, and when they do, it's important to catch them early and appeal quickly.

Don't Rebill, Call!

There are a couple of reasons why. If there's been a mistake on the claims processing end, sending an identical HCFA form risks that the same mistake will be repeated. Due to turnaround time standards and high employee turnover, the pressure may be on the individual claims examiner to churn through an unrealistically high number of claims per day in order to be rated as performing satisfactorily on the job. It's logical that the more speed is emphasized, the more likely it is that accuracy will be compromised. If the response to mistakes is rebilling, this inflates the workload, thus reinforcing the need for speed. The managed care employee can reprocess the claim, avoiding the need to send a duplicate copy. Reprocessing generally works to the therapist's advantage:

Pressure may be on the individual claims examiner to churn through an unrealistically high number of claims per day in order to be rated as performing satisfactorily on the job.

1. It avoids time, hassle, and expense of resubmitting the same claim.
2. It takes less time to get paid.
3. The person who took the phone call is either the one to reprocess the claim, or puts instructions into the computer regarding the correct reprocessing of the claim.

Don't trust that they'll get it right when they reprocess? Document the name of the individual who promised correct reprocessing, and the date on which the conversation occurred. If the claim comes back wrong again, file a formal appeal in writing using that employee's name.

When to Rebill

The one situation where rebilling is advantageous is if the claim appears to be lost, and the company has strict timely filing policies. Better to rebill while there's still time, than to be denied with this as the reason, and all because the company lost the original claim. Yes, claims departments do have their share of black holes.

Advanced Getting Paid Strategies

Knowledge is power. Know the rules, set by the state department of insurance, that govern claims processing. Even if a client's specific benefit plan is subject to ERISA, state insurance departments might still have

Know the rules, set by the state department of insurance, that govern claims processing.

legal regulatory authority over the operations of that insurance or managed care company within the state.

Kathleen Desgranges, LCSW, BCD, profiled in Chapter 14 for her expertise in combating fee reductions, keeps a copy of her state's insurance department regulation specifying turnaround times for claims. She reported that when she files a claim with a company that has been slow, she attaches a photocopy of the regulations to the claim. Inevitably, she says, the claim is paid correctly—and on time.

File written complaints with the state's department of insurance against companies that are slow, make errors, lose claims, or engage in other claims-processing shenanigans.

Linda Walker, one of the billing/practice managers interviewed, commented that she does not hesitate to file written complaints with the state's department of insurance against companies that are slow, make errors, lose claims, or engage in other claims-processing shenanigans. A former claims examiner herself, Ms. Walker is certainly in a position to know what works. Complaints to the department of insurance, she says, produce results because the insurance/managed care companies are monitored for numbers of complaints each year.

I also have found that a simple, polite mention or reminder of the rules to the claims examiner or customer service rep usually results in immediate (and correct) reprocessing of denied claims, or a miraculous "finding" of claims that had been "lost." (This strategy also works very well with the various NCQA standards.)

Appealing denied claims and/or complaining about claims payment practices is the one area that isn't likely to cause a professional to be negatively profiled. It's not typically counted as a measure of managed care friendliness, because so many practitioners use billing services. From a legal and public relations standpoint, the potential consequences of penalizing a therapist who was appropriately following established procedure to get claims paid would likely be much worse to the company than forking over the money. Nor is complaining likely to affect referrals; claims examiners rarely interact with the clinicians and customer service staff who make the referrals.

14

The Finances of Managed Care

Balance Billing

Every managed care contract in existence specifically prohibits balance billing, the practice of billing the client for the portion denied by the managed care company. Another form of balance billing is the practice of billing the client for the difference between the therapist's full fee and the managed care discounted rate. In managed care contracts, this provision is generally found under headings known as exclusive compensation, referring to the first kind of balance billing, and payment in full, referring to the second.

Every managed care contract in existence specifically prohibits balance billing.

While the main idea sounds clear-cut and reasonable enough, in practice things can quickly get tangled, and it's easy for these policies to seem unfair to therapists.

> Carla Rogers had been working with 13-year-old Matt Randall and his family for 6 months. She had been billing their Total Health Insurance plan, which said she was "out-of-network" and paid 50 percent of "usual and customary" after the high deductible was met. The plan allowed 30 outpatient sessions per year for an "out-of-network" provider. Matt's family paid the rest, up to Carla's full fee of $110 per session. Unbeknownst to Carla and the family, THI used the GenRUs Behavioral Health network for their "in-network" mental health benefits, and the GBH case management team for utilization review. Matt's "in-network" mental health benefit plan was structured such that there was no deductible, a $10 copay, and they were entitled to a 50 session per year maximum.
>
> In the seventh month of therapy, GBH completed Carla's credentialing and she became a "participating-provider." Matt's claims began to be denied due to "lack of authorization." Carla's billing service, upon inquiring, was informed that "Dr. Rogers is in-network and should have gotten authorization from GBH." GBH began an authorization for current sessions but refused to grant retro-authorization to cover two months' worth of denied sessions.

THI and GBH, furthermore, ruled that the Randalls were responsible only for $10 per session, and Carla was no longer allowed to charge the family the remainder of her fee. She lost $800 on sessions provided in good faith.

By the terms of her contract with GBH, she received only $60 per session on future sessions when they were authorized as medically necessary, and was expected to discount the remaining $50 of her fee.

What should Carla and her biller do? Nobody's really at fault; when Carla started seeing the Randalls, she was not a part of the GBH network. If Carla bills the Randalls for the insurance company's portion of the sessions that were denied, GBH would consider it balance billing. She and her biller should, instead, file a written appeal, but there isn't much chance of success, since the managed care company would argue that the biller should have investigated the "in-network" benefits and told Carla to obtain authorization when her participating-provider status was finalized.

Therapists should have their client agreements reviewed by an attorney who is familiar with the terms of all contracts they have signed.

Many therapists have included in their intake agreements a provision stating that the client agrees to pay if the insurance denies. While this is appropriate for an out-of-network situation, or for noncovered services, it's very often a contract violation for therapists participating on managed care panels. Therapists should have their client agreements reviewed by an attorney who is familiar with the terms of all contracts they have signed.

Not sure whether a particular situation would be construed as balance billing? Check the contract, the Provider Manual, or consult with an attorney. Or, when in doubt, . . . DON'T.

Waiving Copayments

A pattern of waiving the copayments and/or systemic failure to attempt collection of copayments is one of the things auditors will look for.

Don't do it. If there is ever an audit, a pattern of waiving the copayments and/or systemic failure to attempt collection of copayments is one of the things auditors will look for, and discovery of such a tendency could lead to serious legal trouble with the insurance or managed care company. Why?

Copayments are the insurance/managed care industry's way of providing a built-in disincentive to accessing treatment. The higher the copayment, so the thinking goes, the greater the disincentive for clients to enter or continue in therapy. It makes sense. Think about the increasing popularity of *graduated copayment scales,* benefit formulas that call for the patient to pay a lower copayment in the early sessions, then gradually increase the amount of the copayment until the yearly maximum number of sessions is reached. They're inconvenient and a pain to remember for the client, the therapist, and the therapist's billing/office staff. Not at all inconvenient to the insurance company, if it helps the client make the decision that he or she has had enough treatment. Therapists who waive client copayments are removing the insurance company's disincentive to continue in therapy.

Insurance companies also view writing off copayments as fraudulent. Forgiving a copayment means, to the insurance company, that the therapist is willing to work for less than the contracted fee. If that's the case, then the company's perspective is that the contracted rate should thus be reduced to the level the therapist is willing to accept per session, but preserving the client's copayment portion. In general, insurance companies consider it fraudulent if a therapist is willing to settle for less than the fee billed.

Note that the same holds true if the client owes coinsurance rather than a copayment. Writing off the client's portion, regardless of whether it is a proportion of the contracted fee or a fixed amount, is bad practice.

Out-of-Network Benefits

For practitioners who are not members of managed care networks, the no balance billing rule gets turned on its head: balance billing is expected. It's the same reasoning as why copayments/coinsurance shouldn't be waived: the amount in Box 24-F of the HCFA form is what the therapist should expect to collect. In the absence of a managed care contract binding a practitioner to a discounted contracted rate with exclusive compensation, the client must pay whatever the insurance/managed care company doesn't, or it's considered fraudulent.

For practitioners who are not members of managed care networks, the no balance billing rule gets turned on its head: balance billing is expected.

Isn't there a way to give a client a break? While therapists are certainly free to lower their fees, when an insurance company is involved—even on an out-of-network basis—professionals must honestly report the reduction. If they do not, it is considered insurance fraud, and criminal charges might result if discovered by an auditor.

Cecilia Whitaker, LMFT, was tired of having people express interest in working with her, only to go elsewhere because she didn't belong to managed care networks. She decided that she would lower her fees so that clients would pay no more for seeing her than they would for seeing an in-network therapist.

Mike, the next client to call, had his benefits managed through GBH, and a copay of $20 per session for an in-network therapist. His out-of-network benefits were 50 percent of usual and customary.

Cecilia offered to see Mike, bill GBH her usual fee of $100, and she would consider as payment in full whatever GBH paid her plus $20 per session from Mike.

Cecilia is representing to GBH that whatever they don't pay of that $100, she will bill Mike the difference. Instead, she's writing all but $20 of it off. To an insurance or managed care company, that's fraudulently inflating the charge for the session to get money out of them. If Cecilia wanted to give Mike a discount that was not considered fraudulent, she would have to represent her fee as being what she was willing to take. Thus, if GBH paid 50 percent of $70 usual and customary, or $35, and Mike paid $20, she would have to bill GBH $55. If she did that, GBH would only pay 50 percent of the $55, and Mike would still have an out-of-pocket expense of greater than the $20 in-network copayment.

Insurance companies have a lot of power to define therapists' financial practices, even for professionals who are out-of-network.

It is a misconception that out-of-network means that a therapist is free of insurance and/or managed care.

It is a misconception that out-of-network means that a therapist is free of insurance and/or managed care. Any time an insurance company pays *any* money toward a client's bill, the insurance/managed care company *is* involved and has legally established their right to dictate policies and conduct audits. Being out-of-network is *not* a protection against being audited.

The in-network or out-of-network status of the therapist and the resulting level of benefits paid simply reflects whether the therapist has signed a contract with the insurance/managed care entity.

Sliding Scales, Self-Pay Patients, and the Perils of Setting Fees

It's not just using out-of-network benefits that poses a problem for the therapist in terms of avoiding charges of insurance fraud. Self-pay carries similar issues and risks, because a pattern of systematically charging clients differently for the same service based on their insurance coverage (or lack thereof), is also looked on as fraudulent by insurance companies, and for the same reason. In their eyes, therapists who are willing to take less for some clients should be willing to take less for them all. Therefore, practitioners who receive any kind of reimbursement from private insurance, managed care companies, Blue Cross/Blue Shield, Medicare or Medicaid, must be very careful to avoid any appearance of treating clients differently based on insurance status. The only escape is a 100 percent cash-pay practice.

What about clients who don't have insurance, or whose insurance doesn't cover mental health care, or who have used up their benefits? Working in mental health, we see a lot of sad stories. Many people are in need of treatment, but either don't have insurance, or don't have insurance that will pay. The tradition in mental health treatment has been to modify fees according to the client's ability to pay. In other words, to offer a *sliding scale*.

Is it even possible to have a sliding scale in this day and age? Bart Bernstein, a Dallas attorney specializing in mental health issues, is of the opinion that sliding scales are still possible. The key, though, is meticulous documentation—not a solution that appeals to most of us! Therapists using a sliding scale, says Bernstein, must make it abundantly clear in documentation that the chosen fee is a result of consideration of multiple financial factors, not simply the presence or absence of an insurance policy and what that policy does or doesn't pay (Bernstein & Hartsell, 1998). For example, the therapist might note any significant outstanding debt, a general look at the client's expense/income ratio, and so on. This gets into some complicated procedural questions, such as which factors to consider, and how to document this process appropriately. It also may not be clinically therapeutic. Having worked as a therapist intern in a family service agency that had a formal sliding scale and required each client to fill out a thorough personal financial profile, it's easy to attest to the fact that these proceedings and documentation make clients (and therapists) feel uncomfortable. It might even seem demeaning to the client; no one wants to feel like a charity case. However, documentation (and a good attorney) is essential if therapists ever need to prove that they have not systematically been reducing fees for self-pay clients.

Why is it such an issue? How can it be wrong to give a break to those in need? Well, it's certainly not morally wrong. But the law is not always a

A pattern of systematically charging clients differently for the same service based on their insurance coverage (or lack thereof), is also looked on as fraudulent by insurance companies.

Therapists using a sliding scale must make it abundantly clear in documentation that the chosen fee is a result of consideration of multiple financial factors, not simply the presence or absence of an insurance policy and what that policy does or doesn't pay.

true mirror of morality. In this case, it's necessary to insist on the moral-legal distinction. Everyone knows the story of Robin Hood, and most can agree that robbing the rich to redistribute to the poor, although morally honorable, was legally wrong. The issue of fee discounts to self-pay clients is merely a more complex variation on the same classic theme.

Keep in mind, says Bernstein, that laws can and do change, and that much of healthcare litigation is in its infancy. "The judicial history is short and scattered because this whole problem is less than 5 years old. . . . The last word has not been written on sliding scales."

Cash Discounts

It's a popular trend to give discounts on fees to clients who pay up front and in cash. After all, this considerably reduces a therapist's administrative overhead. It certainly seems reasonable and fair to pass these savings on to the client. However, given the other considerations just discussed, therapists who take *any* insurance reimbursement, governmental or private, of any kind, should consult their attorney before engaging in a practice of standard discounts for cash-payers, or any other group of clients.

Considerations in Setting a Published Fixed Fee

One potential solution for those practitioners not able to document a sliding scale fee is to set a fixed, published rate. It's then generally recommended that this full fee be the charge entered in Box 24-F of every single claim submitted, regardless of whether the practitioner is in or out of the network of that particular insurance or managed care company.

When setting fees, think about the kind of community in which you practice. Does it tend to be a working-class neighborhood? Are the residents highly educated? What are the average income levels? Who are the major employers, and how generously do they pay? Then, consider the kinds of clients you treat. What kinds of financial considerations do they typically have? Clinical specialties might be an important consideration. For example, a therapist specializing in helping women victims of abusive relationships and domestic violence will encounter women who typically have high legal bills (getting divorced, custody fights, etc.), they may not be receiving the child support to which they are entitled, and so on. It would stand to reason that this therapist's full fee might need to be more modest, to accommodate these clients.

While the desire to fall beyond the highest level of usual and customary is understandable for obtaining maximum insurance reimbursement, have a care not to set full fee so high that it is out of affordability range for the majority of self-payers or those for whose insurance you are out-of-network. If the fee has been set at a moderate level, there will be fewer temptations to offer discounts that could lead to a pattern of trouble. Then, consider accepting credit cards and/or working out a payment plan (which must be documented) as ways to help clients who cannot afford to write a check for the remainder every single session.

But be careful! Jean Thoensen, of PsychBiller, LLC, cautions professionals who take Medicare, Medicaid, and/or CHAMPUS patients that technically, "federal law requires that the fees charged to these patients be the lowest fee *customarily* offered to all patients." Note that this requirement does not apply to managed care contracts where the fee schedule may be below Medicare's; these are not customary fees, but contracted ones.

A note about informed consent: Therapists should explain to clients who are planning to use out-of-network benefits, or who will pay the bill themselves and then submit for reimbursement, about the concept of usual and customary, and the expectation that the client will be responsible for whatever insurance doesn't pay, up to the full fee.

While the desire to fall beyond the highest level of usual and customary is understandable for obtaining maximum insurance reimbursement, have a care not to set full fee so high that it is out of affordability range for the majority of self-payers or those for whose insurance you are out-of-network.

Per-Session Fees: The Basic Economic Principles of Supply and Demand

National or regional aggregate fee data, such as the figures reported on the Therapist Insurer Profile web site (see Appendix), or in annual surveys appearing in professional publications, tends to cover up the local variations caused by supply and demand. There's no under-emphasizing just how much the local market affects the fees managed care will pay. The degree of penetration of a particular company in an area is vitally important (and raises antitrust concerns). Companies controlling a sizable proportion of insured lives in a city (figures of 30 to 40 percent are starting to occur as an effect of mergers and acquisitions, particularly on the medical side) are in a position of considerable power. If the fictional GenRUs Behavioral Health administers the behavioral health benefits of 35 percent of all those with insurance in a particular city, GBH is going to have a greater inducement to get local practitioners to accept lower fees than if they only had 5 percent of the insured lives.

There's no under-emphasizing just how much the local market affects the fees managed care will pay.

Penetration of All Managed Care Companies

It's not just the market presence of one company which is a factor; the level of penetration of managed care in general which will drive the fees down. If, for example, only 30 percent of the insureds in a city have managed care, and the rest are still in indemnity plans or nonmanaged PPOs, the managed care companies will have to compete to maintain a reasonable number of network participants by offering better fees than they might otherwise do. However, as the proportion of enrollment in managed care or HMO plans starts to climb, the reimbursements can freely fall. Although it has not yet been proved in a court of law that there is collusion between managed care companies to reduce fees, it does seem to happen that when one major company reduces their rates, the others follow.

Area Quirks

The professional and economic landscape of an area can also have its impact on fees. The sheer number of professionals in an area can drive down the rates; the supply-demand equation has two sides to it. But there can also be other factors. The presence of a single dominant employer, strict state regulation, a famous treatment center, a local hospital chain or dominant group practice that controls the bulk of the medical/behavioral health treatment, can all impact reimbursements, for good or for ill.

Controlling Our Numbers

The question on everyone's lips is "How low can the fees go?" Unfortunately, the field doesn't seem to have "hit bottom" just yet. According to Kirk Griffith, PhD, senior vice president of Clinical Network Management at Magellan Behavioral Health, "the fundamental challenge for the field right now is the issue of oversupply of providers. There's no getting around that, and it creates a real macro-economic pressure."

The fundamental challenge for the field right now is the issue of oversupply of providers.

How bad is it? Bad, and likely to get worse. The industry newsletter Open Minds reported in September 1997 that on average, there are 114 behavioral health professionals per 100,000 members of the population (Mills, 1997). The study they were referring to, conducted by Brett Steenbarger, PhD, of the Department of Psychiatry at SUNY—Syracuse, counted psychiatrists, psychologists, social workers, professional counselors, marriage and family therapists, and certified nurse specialists.

However, Steenbarger concluded that only about 70 professionals per 100,000 population would be a balanced proportion. And there's still more to come, currently enrolled in the graduate schools of all disciplines.

Rural practice is an option. In rural areas where there are no network participants, the typical practice is to pay as billed. The managed care company's loss through occasionally paying a rural clinician's full fee is more than covered by all the discounted rates to the rest of us in the cities and suburbs. So should therapists become like that doctor on the television show "Northern Exposure" and relocate to the frozen wilderness of Cicely, Alaska? After all, how much work can there be in very thinly populated areas? It's hard to say. There are many personal as well as professional factors involved in a decision about where to locate and establish a practice.

In rural areas where there are no network participants, the typical practice is to pay as billed.

How does it work for these lucky few? The former Network Development manager who was interviewed indicated that "there was no fee negotiation unless a therapist was needed in the area." So, for example, the only psychiatrist within a 2-hour drive can determine what fees he or she will and won't accept from managed care, and the managed care company has little choice in the matter. The advantage of being a lone wolf in a rural or semi-rural area can apply to specialties as well as disciplines. Even being one of just a handful can be advantageous if there is a high level of need, such as for board-certified child/adolescent psychiatrists.

Exception: Public Sector

If the government sets the rates, then the supply-and-demand dynamic doesn't hold true, regardless of the inherent advantages of an under-served region. Just be careful to read the contract; there's no reason to agree to low rates for all business, just to be able to serve the Medicaid population.

Will technology obliterate rural professionals' negotiating power altogether? Although the possibility of tele-services to members in rural areas is being discussed, and there are some experiments being conducted by different companies (*Managed Care Strategies*, April 1999), this trend has not firmly taken hold yet. Ethical and legal issues complicate the delivery of services in settings which are not face-to-face: how would the tele-practitioner intervene in a crisis situation? Can a psychiatrist monitor medications effectively (or even prescribe to begin with) in a tele-services setting? Until these issues are worked out, supply and demand economics

The law of supply and demand, and the managed care company's past experience, says that for each therapist who won't accept low rates, there will be another who will.

will clearly continue to favor professionals who choose to practice in rural areas.

Being one of many, the power is theirs. Just ask any younger therapist struggling to start a private practice and hearing over and over again that panels are closed in their urban or suburban zip codes. The law of supply and demand, and the managed care company's past experience, says that for each therapist who won't accept low rates, there will be another who will. This fact alone is often what keeps therapists in the managed care panels.

Straddling the Fence

Many therapists argue that fee reductions cause a decline in the quality of the professionals remaining on the panels, asserting that only inexperienced practitioners stay on panels until they can establish their practices. Intuitive though that may seem, unfortunately there's only anecdotal data available at this time to support or refute this claim. When asked, Dr. Griffith of Magellan commented, "We haven't seen any trends in the data with regard to who has resigned in response to fee cuts. The numbers who have resigned over fees is tiny. . . . We hear the concern but data don't support it." The functional disenrollment phenomenon, where clinicians stay on panels but attempt take only a limited number of managed care referrals at any one time, supports Dr. Griffith's conclusion. If practitioners remain on panels, then of course it looks as if the managed care company can reduce fees with little impact on the quality or quantity of the professionals on the network.

How low are the companies going to try to push the fees? Who knows? For the moment, practitioners cannot legally join forces to collectively bargain with insurance companies. However, as individuals, each of us can do something about it.

Challenging Fee Reductions

It is possible, with the right strategy and enough persistence, according to Kathleen Desgranges, LCSW, BCD, of Grand Blanc, Michigan. Ms. Desgranges has successfully challenged five major insurers over fee reductions and other policy decisions adversely affecting her practice. Kathleen Desgranges practices with her sister, a child psychiatrist, and another practitioner, a PhD, in an incorporated group specializing in children and adolescents. She estimates that at least 70 percent of her group's patients use insurance, and that the community in which she practices, a suburb of Flint, "is as overflowing with therapists as most other places."

The Method

Kathleen Desgranges likes to refer to her method and philosophy as "Go ahead, nibble a little: How to effectively bite the hand that feeds you." She begins with these basic premises:

1. We will not let ourselves become dependent on any one company's referrals, to such an extent that it would be the ruin of us if they stopped referring or if we had to resign from the panel.
2. Through JCAHO accreditation, our practice has demonstrated value in terms of quality services, ability to live up to standards of treatment planning, documentation, and cost-effective treatment.

Our practice has demonstrated value.

3. It is important to turn adversarial situations into collaborative ones. Objecting to rates or policies must be done in a professional manner to be effective.
4. Being assertive about the fees and policies which affect our practice is a must, no matter how much time it takes to write letters and make phone calls. Reimbursement rates must be sufficient to allow us to stay in business.
5. Employers do care about the quality of services provided to employees, and as an advocate for patients I am acting honestly and ethically in informing employers when the managed care companies they hire are making conditions impossible for quality services to be performed.

Kathleen Desgranges' most recent struggle, in the fall of 1998, when a major insurer announced rate cuts for 1999, is a typical example of how things play out using her methods. She responded to the initial announcement immediately in writing, objecting firmly to the rate reduction (Figure 14.1). Immediately, meant within one week of receiving the notice. Although she probably was just as angry as anyone else, she did not allow complaining to interfere with taking action. There's not much time allowed by contracts to object to fee reductions (see Chapter 4).

Figure 14.1
Letter Objecting to Rate Reductions

[date]
[name & title]
[company]
[address]
[city, state, zip]

Re: Your proposed reimbursement for social work services

Dear [name],

Last week we received your 1999 and future contract for services to [name of employer]'s employees and their dependents. After living through the past several years, each of which included significant increases in costs of doing business, I was appalled to see that you are proposing a 22% reduction in reimbursement for services rendered by clinical social workers. When I called to seek some understanding of this, I was advised that your company thought this was a fair and equitable reimbursement rate.

Perhaps you are unaware of the costs of doing business. We have been accredited by the Joint Commission on Accreditation of Health Care Organizations for over 10 years. We maintain compliance with the standards of care at a level that has given this agency accreditation with commendation the last two surveys and before that we were listed in the top 10% of agencies (before there was commendation). We were last surveyed last week and received 1's in all areas with no recommendations for improvement of services or management of the facility. We anticipate another accreditation with commendation. We would be happy to sit down with "the powers that be" and look at how we should cut this unnecessary fat out of our budget, as we are running at margin and have been for the past several years. There is no profit, nor are there large salaries. Feel free to come and look at what expenses must be met.

Perhaps you feel all Clinical Social Workers should have their income reduced by this figure. Have you also reduced the salaries of all clinical case managers on this program a commensurate amount?

Perhaps you believe the proposed rates make you competitive with other companies. Of the contracts we hold, you will be reimbursing at a rate significantly below the following [lists 18 companies by name]. It is true, your proposed reimbursement level is above that of [lists two companies by name]. This does not strike me as the way you wish to be regarded among the mental health professionals. Is it really?

I realize you may argue that the social work rate was reduced to allow you to enhance the payment level of psychiatrists. However, we all know the two professions are not providing services in equal amounts and therefore, this plan to rob from one group to enhance another does not even make sense. It appears arbitrary and discriminatory to my profession.

Please contact me at your earliest convenience to review my concerns and allow me to better understand how to manage the clinical services here at a seriously reduced rate of reimbursement.

Sincerely,

Kathleen Desgranges

Source: Reprinted with permission of Kathleen Desgranges, LCSW, BCD.

The Desgranges letter is effectively written for a number of reasons, all of which correspond to her stated method:

1. The tone is polite, professional, and collaborative. There's no angry "you're all a bunch of greedy bloodsucking bastards making a disgraceful profit on our backs" rhetoric.
2. The letter highlights the value of Desgranges' practice in terms of maintaining quality standards, and does so in a way that the managed care company can't refute or discount (JCAHO accreditation).
3. As the cornerstone of her argument about maintaining quality, Desgranges highlights the crucial link with cost: Quality must be paid for.
4. The letter refutes the stated reason about needing to reduce rates to stay competitive, and shows the company exactly where their proposed new rates place them. In the actual letter, Desgranges mentioned the competitor company names, but did not reveal what the competitors' level of reimbursement was.

Quality must be paid for.

The paragraph about psychiatrists was there in response to the specific stated nature of this particular fee reduction, which was an unbundling of services provided by groups, with a slight increase in the reimbursement rates for psychiatrists but a corresponding dramatic decrease in the rates for social workers. For the most part, the letter takes a logical, rational look at each of the arguments the insurance company might use regarding their decision to lower the fees, and calmly explains why these are not valid.

Notice that Kathleen does not threaten to resign; it would not serve her purpose to do so. Why not? Practitioner oversupply. Those numbers give managed care companies the ability to take the attitude of "there's more where you came from." Threatening resignation would not only be meaningless to a managed care company, it might actually even serve their purposes, because then they would not have to deal with an assertive professional, like Kathleen Desgranges, who stands up for his or her rights. Instead of threatening to resign, Desgranges highlights her contribution to the quality of the network in a way that managed care can appreciate.

Practitioner oversupply. Those numbers give managed care companies the ability to take the attitude of "there's more where you came from."

The letter is just the first step. Not surprisingly, the response to Desgranges' letter was a standard "Dear Provider" form letter acknowledging receipt of her objections and restating the original reasons for the fee reduction. Some companies have been known not to respond for quite a while, if at all. Regardless of whether a response is received, the Desgranges method involves persistent follow-up to the original objection letter.

Keep climbing the corporate ladder. Start with Provider Relations, advises Desgranges, and work upward. Ask who is in charge of making the decisions about reimbursement rates, and ask to speak to that person. It may be necessary to get firm. (I can attest to the fact that those higher up the corporate ladder expect those below to protect them from annoying phone calls.) Desgranges has a piece of useful advice when being stonewalled by a low-level employee. Simply say, in as nice a tone as possible, "You mean you're refusing to let me speak with your supervisor?" or, "You mean you're refusing to give me the name of the person in charge?" When put like that, it forces the employee's hand. But if for some reason they continue to refuse to transfer her, Desgranges takes the employee's name, then hangs up and calls back. Eventually, she gets where she is bound.

The Desgranges method involves persistent follow-up to the original objection letter.

Getting the Ear of the Employer

Kathleen Desgranges is firm on one very important point: she refuses to involve clients in this process. It is not appropriate to triangulate clients or expect them to violate their own confidentiality by asking that they complain to their employer or help therapists find the proper person within their company. Instead, she makes cold calls to the affected employer(s)' Human Resources Department. What she asks is who negotiated the contract with the managed care company? Or, who is the liaison with the managed care company?

It is not appropriate to triangulate clients or expect them to violate their own confidentiality by asking that they complain to their employer or help therapists find the proper person within their company.

Desgranges admits that less assertive individuals might find this difficult. "Nobody has ever accused me of being unassertive," she says. But, she advises, believing in the cause helps. After all, the person on the other end of the phone might be in need of help one day and want to use their benefits to obtain it. Despite managed care companies' assertions that quality professionals aren't leaving networks in any significant numbers due to fee reductions, those in charge of benefits administration, hearing the facts as laid out in the Desgranges letter, will become concerned.

Be prepared to repeat the story to several people. Often, the first few people don't know who is the correct person for Desgranges to speak with. So, she simply accepts to be transferred to the most likely candidate, taking the opportunity at each step to share the story. Revealing the facts of the situation, even to lower-level HR administrators, often causes enough consternation and talk in the department that the right person hears about it and comes to Desgranges. "They're receptive because they want to make sure their employees get good service. They recognize that a 22 percent fee cut means the best people will drop out of the network." Inevitably, she says, the managed care company's customers never know about the fee reductions until she informs them.

Usually, this is all it takes. "Calling the companies has tremendous weight. One or two phone calls from the employer and the insurance company buckles," says Desgranges.

Don't you get blacklisted? I asked Kathleen Desgranges about the typical response of managed care companies after they have agreed not to reduce her contracted fees. Desgranges admits that for a time, referrals do stop, but it's almost always temporary. In fact, she and her sister once sued Blue Cross of Michigan, yet two years later the company approached the Desgranges practice to serve on their panel.

"They're receptive because they want to make sure their employees get good service. They recognize that a 22 percent fee cut means the best people will drop out of the network."

15

Putting the Money at Risk

The fundamental ethical dilemma of risk-based methods of reimbursement stems from the fact that the practitioner is paid more for offering less treatment.

The nature of insurance is risk. In its simplest form, insurance of any type collects a pool of money from premiums and gambles that the number of people who stay healthy, who avoid car accidents, whose houses don't burn down, and so on, will remain small enough such that reimbursing their losses/medical bills won't exhaust the pool. Anything left over is profit. Managed care and managed behavioral care companies do it too, in the form of at-risk contracts (see Chapter 7).

Professionals are being asked to take the same risk in new models of reimbursement. These risk-based reimbursement methods, known as case rates and capitation, have engendered quite a bit of controversy. Capitation refers to a population of "covered lives," whereas case rates are for one client only. The fundamental ethical dilemma of the risk-based methods of reimbursement stems from the fact that the practitioner is paid more for offering less treatment.

Case Rates: (De)Capitating the Single Therapist

A case rate is a lump-sum payment for each individual case, regardless of the number of sessions the client needs to be seen, up to the number of sessions pre-determined by the client's employer or benefit plan. Employee assistance programs frequently use case rates, since the maximum number of EAP sessions is predetermined anyway. When used for managed care benefits, case rates are defined as a certain sum paid to the therapist to cover anywhere from one to a prespecified number of sessions (usually 8–12). No medical necessity utilization review is conducted during the block of sessions covered by the case rate; it's up to the discretion of the client and the therapist to determine the client's treatment needs and how best to use the sessions.

If all the sessions are used and the client continues to need treatment, there is usually an outpatient treatment report or phone review with a case manager, just as if the therapist had been paid on a per-session basis. Typically, once the maximum number of sessions on the original case rate has been reached, the reimbursement then reverts to the therapist's discounted per-session contracted fee, because at this point it has been established that the client needs longer term therapy, and placing reimbursement at-risk would not be appropriate.

Calculating the Case Rates

It's not uncommon to hear therapists at conferences, or in casual conversation, say, "*I wouldn't necessarily mind a case rate, if they would just set the case rate figure to what would be a reasonable per-session fee.*" Whether or not a specific dollar amount is unreasonable or inadequate may be very true, but this comment misses the whole point of the case rate, which is to:

1. Save the managed care company money and staff time by reducing the need for utilization review.
2. Further incentivize the use of short-term, solution-focused care.
3. Reduce the managed care company's liability for denying authorization.

The managed care organization which offers case rates is gambling that the client will use at least as many sessions as the $200 to $300 would cover under a fee-for-service model, if not more. The company loses money if they pay a therapist a $250 case rate and the client is seen only once or twice. But by paying the therapist up front, the managed care company gains these three advantages. The balancing out effect is the key to case rates. There will be cases in which the client is seen only once and the company pays more per session than if they had offered a discounted per-session fee, but there will also be cases in which the therapist uses the maximum number of sessions and the company pays less per session than they would have done with a fee-for-service model.

The balancing out effect is the key to case rates.

Surviving and Thriving with Case Rates

Survival is possible, but it requires a change of mindset, without which one should probably not accept a case rate agreement. Therapists who

Case rates require a volume of clients before one can make any meaningful conclusions about what a therapist is really earning on a per-session basis.

Therapists who are successful with case rates exclusively practice brief, solution-oriented therapy.

are successful with case rates have moved beyond the tendency to do what all of us do, at least initially; namely, to mentally break down the case rate, after the client has been discharged, into what was ultimately paid on a per session basis. Case rates require a volume of clients before one can make any meaningful conclusions about what a therapist is really earning on a per-session basis. All one or two cases will demonstrate is that the therapist either scored big financially or lost money on the deal. Therapists who do well with case rates are those who have adopted the long-term risk management mindset: do the clients who only come in once or twice effectively balance the ones who need to be seen for the full 6, 8, or 10 sessions?

And of course, it practically goes without saying that therapists who are successful with case rates exclusively practice brief, solution-oriented therapy. It requires being comfortable with discharging the client after the immediate presenting problem is resolved. Even for therapists who are relatively comfortable with short-term models of therapy, this is not an easy thing to do.

Determining Whether Accepting a Case Rate Is a Good Move

There is a way to get an idea of whether one will be successful, prior to signing the contract. Go back over the last 100 discounted fee-for-service insurance or managed care clients who were discharged. How many times were each of these clients seen?

With this data, it's possible to evaluate a proposed case rate. Let's say the managed care company is offering a case rate of $300 for up to 10 sessions. By looking at a minimum of the last hundred clients, it's possible to calculate what would have been earned had each of these clients been using this case rate plan. Begin by noting how many clients discharged after the first session, second, third, and so on, going all the way up to 10. Since after 10 sessions under the proposed case rate, clients would switch over to per-session fees, log the number of clients who had more than 10 sessions as "10." Table 15.1 shows the calculations.

It's possible to repeat these calculations with the last 200 clients, or 500, or as many as are available. In general, the larger the sample, the more accurate the calculations, and the less the average will be thrown off by a client who is seen only once or all 10 times.

Table 15.1

Sample Case Rate Adequacy Calculations (Assumes last 100 clients, a case rate of $300 for up to 10 sessions)

10 sessions	+	35 clients	$300 each × 35 = $10500 / 350 sessions	=	$30 per session
9 sessions		7 clients	$300 each × 7 = $2100 / 63 sessions	=	$33.33 per session
8 sessions		9 clients	$300 each × 9 = $2700 / 72 sessions	=	$37.5 per session
7 sessions		6 clients	$300 each × 6 = $1800 / 42 sessions	=	$42.86 per session
6 sessions		5 clients	$300 each × 5 = $1500 / 30 sessions	=	$50 per session
5 sessions		14 clients	$300 each × 14 = $4200 / 70 sessions	=	$60 per session
4 sessions		2 clients	$300 each × 2 = $600 / 8 sessions	=	$75 per session
3 sessions		5 clients	$300 each × 5 = $1500 / 15 sessions	=	$100 per session
2 sessions		4 clients	$300 each × 4 = $1200 / 8 sessions	=	$150 per session
1 session:		13 clients	$300 each × 13 = $3900 / 13 sessions	=	$300 per session

1. The per-session rate is not affected by how many clients were seen that number of times. In other words, no matter how many clients are seen for 5 sessions, the per-session rate will always equal $60.

2. The adequacy of the case rate is determined by the distribution of how many times the population of clients was seen. To figure this, divide the total amount paid by the total number of sessions.

100 clients × $300 each = $30,000 total amount paid

$30,000 / 671 sessions = $44.71 per session

Average number of sessions per client = 6.71

Is this figure high enough to cover expenses, taxes, and profit, assuming similar utilization patterns?

In Table 15.1, the average number of sessions per client, 6.71, was a bit high. Let's say that the average number of sessions was only 4.76 per client. This would increase the profitability of the case rate, to $63 per session. Hence, the ethical dilemma—and the risk—involved in this kind of reimbursement method.

Relationships with case managers at the EAP/managed care company do tend to differ according to the reimbursement arrangements. When the reimbursement is a case rate system, case managers are instructed to monitor therapists for underutilization; with per-session fees, it's the opposite. Expect questions or challenges from the case manager not when more sessions are requested under a case rate, but when the client is referred after only one or two sessions. Provider-profiling under a case rate system also looks at average numbers of sessions per client, but the sessions-per-case average is interpreted in exactly the opposite manner from when the therapist is paid on a per-session basis.

A few therapists, particularly with EAP case rates, openly say that their strategy is to see the client once or twice and then refer. This is unethical,

When the reimbursement is a case rate system, case managers are instructed to monitor therapists for underutilization; with per-session fees, it's the opposite.

and unfair to the clients, some of whom might be able to achieve some benefit from short-term therapy up to the maximum number of sessions permitted. Furthermore, it's likely to cause trouble for the therapist in the end. Accepting a case rate contract arrangement with the intention of referring all or most clients as soon as possible will eventually result in client complaints, negative profiling, and/or disciplinary action by the managed care company, possibly even a licensing board.

The important thing is to have a firm clinical rationale for every decision made, with case rates as with per-session fees.

Just as therapists make ethical clinical decisions despite the built-in traditional bias of "more sessions = more money," it's possible to do this with case rates. The important thing is to have a firm clinical rationale for every decision made, with case rates as with per-session fees. If therapists paid on a case rate system can verbalize this rationale to case managers (who will document it in the managed care company's computer system), there should not be a problem.

Capitation

A capitated contract counts heads and pays on that basis.

In return for prepayment based on enrollment in the insurance plan, any covered member must be seen at any time, for any medically necessary service covered by the plan—at any level of care.

The word *capitation* comes from the Latin *capita*, meaning head. Literally, a capitated contract counts heads and pays on that basis. Unlike a case rate, it is based on a population of clients. Solo practitioners cannot accept capitated contracts, because in return for prepayment based on enrollment in the insurance plan, any covered member must be seen at any time, for any medically necessary service covered by the plan—at any level of care.

Groups accepting capitated reimbursement systems are paid on a *per-member-per-month* basis, often abbreviated as PMPM. All they collect at the time of service is the patient's copayment. Capitation is also a mainstay of employee assistance programs, and in EAPs, the payment is PEPM—per employee per month—in exchange for any service offered by the EAP (assessment, brief counseling, CISD, management consultations, etc.).

Advantages

Capitation gets rid of the need to file claims. There's no more waiting 60 or 90 days for claims to be paid, or spending time on the phone with the insurance company getting claims straightened out. The group is paid each month and simply reports utilization data to the insurer or managed care company. There's no need to do OTRs for additional sessions; there's no need, in fact, for authorizations from the managed care company at all, so the number of case managers who have to be hired—and paid—by the managed care company is reduced. The group practice itself determines what is medically necessary, using whatever real-life criteria they see fit to adopt.

The Ethical Dilemma

It's the same one faced by managed care companies with at-risk contracts. If too many people need too many costly services, and they all have to be treated even after the money is gone, the group could very easily go bankrupt. And many groups have.

Going Capitated

Aside from the ethical dilemmas, capitation sounds fairly straightforward, but it's not. [Groups] ". . . forget that the contract is for two services—live clinical care and managing mental health services. The manager role is a clearly purchased service," says Gayle Zieman, PhD, author of the *Complete Capitation Handbook* and a veteran of successful negotiation and implementation of capitated contracts. Capitation has raised the stakes well beyond the model of the clinician-small businessperson, or group of collaborating clinicians, that handle all practice matters alone or with the help of a billing service. Doing capitation right means that groups must hire and/or retain people with the necessary business, computer, and legal expertise. Growth and survival of a group practice in a managed care-dominated marketplace is a business enterprise, not a clinical one, and unfortunately relying on the ability to provide good clinical care just isn't enough. Table 15.2 provides a list of the most important practical as well as clinical questions groups need to consider before signing a capitated contract.

[Groups] ". . . forget that the contract is for two services—live clinical care and managing mental health services. The manager role is a clearly purchased service."

Considerations in PMPM Calculations

PMPM rates are no less vulnerable to the current squeeze in reimbursement than are discounted per-session rates to individual contract clinicians (*Managed Care Strategies*, December 1998). And these rates must include *everything*. Unless a group practice *subcapitates* from a larger

Table 15.2
Getting Ready for Capitation

Groups need to study their ability to provide administration of a capitated contract as well as the clinical services. Typical management functions are claims payment, QI/outcomes measurement, network/credentialing, preventive services, and utilization review. Will the insurer/managed care company be putting performance of certain indicators at further risk using a withhold or a rebate method (see Chapter 1)?

- What financial resources does the practice have to withstand periods of utilization that are higher than expected?
- Does the practice have the information systems resources to do the job? If not, how will the purchase of a system be financed, and what will be the training needs of the staff?
- How will intake and triage be handled? Will a separate team be responsible or will practicing clinicians take turns? Consider the costs as well as the impact on quality of care of various options for structuring this service.
- How will after-hours and emergency services be covered? Will there be a separate team or will practicing clinicians take turns? How will these duties be compensated?
- What happens if a member needs a higher level of care or specialty care? Consider the kinds of contractual arrangements the practice has with facilities, medical, and specialty professionals in the community. What kinds of aftercare programs and other wraparound services can the practice offer for clients who need them to maintain functioning after discharge from inpatient or other intensive treatment?
- How will utilization review be handled? Will there be a separate utilization review team or will practicing clinicians take turns? How will utilization review duties be paid for, or worked into clinicians' productivity targets?
- What "medical necessity" criteria will the group use? How will it be developed and implemented? Will best practices guidelines be adopted?
- How will appeals be handled/who will do them? How will they be paid? There will need to be an attorney to make sure that appeals procedures are compliant with applicable law.
- Will the group need to use an independent review organization for final-level appeals?
- Who will perform the QI functions? Separate QI team or practicing clinicians? How will QI duties be paid for/worked into clinicians' productivity targets?
- Does the group currently measure their outcomes, utilization, and patient satisfaction? If not, how will this be implemented? Consider cost factors as well as logistics and clinical value of the various options and measurement tools/strategies.
- Will the managed care company expect the practice to document compliance to NCQA standards/become accredited? How well does the practice currently conform to NCQA standards? What will be needed to improve compliance, how much will this cost, and who will be responsible?
- Does the group currently measure accessibility in terms of appointment wait times? Does accessibility meet NCQA's standards?
- How will the group structure duties so as to use staff in the most efficient and cost-effective manner, but making sure that quality of care is not affected?
- Will the group be required to pay claims for services provided to members outside the practice? Does the group have the infrastructure and knowledge required to pay claims?
- How will the group practice balance the obligations of the capitated contract with its obligations to self-payers and clients using other insurance plans?
- How will the group continue its marketing activities such that the practice doesn't become overly dependent on the capitated contract as its only source of income?
- Do the group's clinicians truly understand and accept the need to adapt practice patterns to fit a capitated practice environment? Are they willing to conduct brief treatment, group therapy, and preventive care?

integrated delivery system to just perform outpatient services, the PMPM has to include medication management, groups, intake/triage and other emergency services, inpatient stays, possibly detoxification, residential, intensive outpatient, partial hospitalization, ECT, psych testing, and any other covered mental health/chemical dependency services (this generally excludes the price of prescription medication). It's whatever is in the contract.

Table 15.2 identifies just how many hidden service-delivery costs there are that can easily cause serious financial problems if not planned and budgeted for. Staff costs and allocation are particularly tricky. Utilization review, appeals, intake, emergency services, and outcomes measurement are all useful and necessary, but to what extent can a group's clinicians be expected to provide them effectively in addition to their main responsibility of treating patients? Workload issues can easily cause serious staff morale problems. Because of the incredibly tight margins under capitation, says Dr. Zieman, the issues of volume and additional responsibilities "become a battle with staff clinicians. The only way to operate in the black is to impose rigorous productivity models." "It's the group version of what happens in solo practice when the managed care companies cut the reimbursement rates but then say, 'Oh, by the way, we want you to fill out this extra form.'" And this is an important reason why groups have not been able to completely eclipse solo practitioners.

Then there will be those instances where members must use services outside the group, but which the group must pay for. The group with a capitated contract pays for *all* medically necessary, covered services to members regardless of who provides the service. Remarked Zieman, "I always tell groups taking cap contracts, YOU WILL have subcontracted providers even if you think you cover all specialties. There are always some services you don't have in-house, and then there are the circumstances that must fall outside your group." Examples of the latter: a member with children in college or who reside with an ex-spouse, and require services in another city where the group does not have operations.

Other Capitation Considerations

Contract Negotiation

The complexities of contract negotiations are beyond the scope of this book, except for some very general advice: get help, do your homework, and don't be afraid to pass on a contract that seems too financially risky. There are technical features of contracts, such as graduated capitation or stop-loss clauses, that can provide some financial safeguards for groups if utilization turns out to be higher than expected. But groups that don't do their homework won't be able to negotiate effectively for what they need to offer quality services. Better to pass on a contract than underbid and provide shoddy care—and/or end up bankrupt. As Dr. Zieman said, quite candidly, "the final bid usually goes to . . . who[ever] says they can do it for the lowest cost. Capitated contracts are won and lost over 1–5¢ PMPM differences. . . . It's hard for groups to be even in the price ballpark of a Magellan or ValueOptions."

Groups that don't do their homework won't be able to negotiate effectively for what they need to offer quality services.

Preventive Care

The theory behind HMOs, in the very beginning, was that more plentiful and cheaper preventive care would reduce the occurrence (and therefore the costs) of more serious illness. In any population of covered individuals, there will be those who will use no services at all, those who use preventive and/or relatively low-cost treatments, and those who, by virtue of being more seriously ill, use significant resources. In a capitated system, the very ill minority can easily use up the majority of the resources, thus eliminating the financial ability of the practice to offer preventive and/or outreach care. Preventive mental health services are no different from preventive medical services, in this regard.

For groups considering capitating or subcapitating mental health and/or substance abuse services, preventive care will undoubtedly be a requirement of the contract. It's an NCQA (1998, 2000) requirement, which the managed care organizations offering the capitated contract have to meet for accreditation. Specifically, NCQA (2000, PH 4) expects that at least two separate prevention programs per year will be implemented. The members and practitioners must be notified of the programs, and the effects of the programs must be measured. Typically, with the exception of notifications, groups accepting capitated contracts become delegates of the managed care company with respect to meeting these standards. This means that groups must consider, prior to signing the contract, what their programs will be, and what will be the costs of these programs. Since the cost for prevention programs must come out of the overall PMPM, it's important to figure in these costs ahead of time. There may or may not be the chance to renegotiate after the contract is signed.

NCQA expects that at least two separate prevention programs per year will be implemented.

NCQA, Accreditation, and the Capitated Group Practice

Although at this time NCQA does not offer accreditation programs for groups and/or integrated delivery systems, it's very likely that over the next three to five years they will. In the meantime, there are several other accreditation organizations, the most prominent being JCAHO, from which groups can seek accreditation. While it may be a headache to obtain, the role of such accreditation is important in demonstrating quality to payors, and there's no reason to expect that this will change in the near future. Kathleen Desgranges' example (see Chapter 14) of maintaining reasonable reimbursement rates depended heavily on the fact that her group was JCAHO-accredited.

For the purposes of NCQA accreditation of managed care organizations, groups accepting capitation are considered delegates. NCQA allows managed care organizations to subcontract, or delegate, most functions (i.e., utilization management, preventive care, etc.) to another organization, such as a group practice, with the stipulation that the managed care company retain oversight (unless the entity accepting delegation is independently NCQA-accredited). This is what Dr. Zieman was referring to when he explained that the manager role is an explicitly purchased service. What this means for the practice is that NCQA's standards must be met by the group if the managed care company is to maintain/obtain accreditation. For a group to document that NCQA's standards are being met requires significant financial investment in information systems and quality assurance personnel—all of which must come out of the PMPM rate.

For a group to document that NCQA's standards are being met requires significant financial investment in information systems and quality assurance personnel—all of which must come out of the PMPM rate.

State Regulation

State regulation goes even beyond the complexities of the capitated contract negotiation process. Because the inherent definition of capitation involves assuming financial risk, state insurance departments may define even a group practice that offers healthcare services under a contract involving financial risk as "insurance." Depending on the state's definition, there may be licensing and/or other operating regulations—even if it's just an EAP contract (*Managed Care Strategies*, March 1999). Insurance companies have to prove that they have enough capital to withstand losses (called a "capitalization requirement"), according to certain formulas derived either by the state's Insurance Department or the National Association of Insurance Commissioners (NAIC). After all, the state Department of Insurance's job is to protect citizens, who may be adversely affected if the group is unable to provide needed services for which the member has already paid a premium. It gets quite technical, so groups pursuing direct contracting must hire a knowledgeable attorney and consult with the officials at their state's Department of Insurance (see Appendix).

Appendix
State Insurance Departments

Alabama

201 Monroe St., Suite 1700
Montgomery, AL 36104
(334) 269-3550

Alaska

http://www.commerce.state.ak.us/insurance/
3601 C Street, Suite 1324
Anchorage, AK 99503-5948
(907) 269-7900

Arizona

http://www.state.az.us/id/
2910 N. 44th Street, Suite 210
Phoenix, AZ 85018
(602) 912-8444 or (800) 325-2548

Arkansas

http://www.state.ar.us/insurance/
1200 W. 3rd Street
Little Rock, AR 72201-1904
(501) 371-2600 or (800) 852-5494

California

http://www.insurance.ca.gov/docs/index.html
300 Capitol Mall, Suite 1500
Sacramento, CA 95814
(916) 492-3500
Department of Corporations regulates health care
  service plans: (800) 400-0815

Colorado

http://www.dora.state.co.us/insurance/consumer/cons
umenu.htm
1560 Broadway, Suite 850
Denver, CO 80202
(303) 894-7499 or (800) 930-3745

Connecticut

http://www.state.ct.us/cid/
P.O. Box 816
Hartford, CT 06142-0816
(860) 297-3802

Delaware

http://www.state.de.us/inscom/index.htm
1st Federal Plaza, 710 North King Street
Wilmington, DE 19801
(302) 577-3119

District of Columbia

441 Fourth St. NW, 8th Floor North
Washington, DC 20001
(202) 727-8000

Florida

http://www.doi.state.fl.us/
200 East Gaines Street
Tallahassee, FL 32399-0300
(850) 922-3100 or (800) 342-2762

Georgia

http://www.InsComm.State.Ga.US/
2 Martin Luther King, Jr. Drive
West Tower, Suite 704
Atlanta, GA 30334
(404) 656-2070 or (800) 656-2298

Hawaii

http://www.state.hi.us/insurance/
250 S. King Street, 5th Floor
Honolulu, HI 96813
(808) 586-2790

Idaho

http://www.doi.state.id.us/
700 West State Street, 3rd Floor
Boise, ID 83720-0043
(208) 334-4250 or (800) 721-3272

Illinois

http://www.state.il.us/ins/consumerinfo.htm
320 W. Washington St., 4th Floor
Springfield, IL 62767-0001
(217) 782-4515 or (217) 782-7446

Indiana

http://www.state.in.us/idoi/
311 West Washington St., Suite 300
Indianapolis, IN 46204-2787
(317) 232-2385 or (800) 622-4461

Iowa

http://www.state.ia.us/government/com/ins/ins.htm
330 E. Maple St.
Des Moines, IA 50319-0065
(515) 281-5705 or (515) 281-4241

Kansas

http://www.ink.org/public/kid/
420 Southwest Ninth St.
Topeka, KS 66612-1678
(785) 296-3071, (800) 432-2484, or (800) 860-5260

Kentucky

http://www.doi.state.ky.us/
215 West Main Street
Frankfort, KY 40601
(502) 564-3630, (502) 564-6004, or (800) 595-6053

Louisiana

http://www.ldi.state.la.us/
950 N. Fifth St.
Baton Rouge, LA 70804-9214
(225) 342-5900, (800) 259-5300, or (800) 259-5301

Maine

http://www.state.me.us/pfr/ins/inshome2.htm
34 State House Station
Augusta, ME 04333
(207) 624-8475 or (800) 300-5000

Maryland

http://www.gacc.com/mia/
525 St. Paul Place
Baltimore, MD 21202
(410) 468-2000 or (800) 492-6116

Massachusetts

http://www.magnet.state.ma.us/doi/
470 Atlantic Avenue, 6th Floor
Boston, MA 02210-2223
(617) 521-7794 or (800) 436-7757

Michigan

http://www.commerce.state.mi.us/ins/pageone.htm
611 West Ottawa St., 2nd Floor North
Lansing, MI 48933
(517) 373-9273

Minnesota

http://www.commerce.state.mn.us/mainin.htm
133 E. 7th St.
St. Paul, MN 55101
(612) 296-6848

Mississippi

http://www.doi.state.ms.us/
1804 Walter Sillers Bldg.
550 High Street
Jackson, MS 39201
(601) 359-3569 or (800) 562-2957

Missouri

http://www.insurance.state.mo.us/
P.O. Box 690
Jefferson City, MO 65102-0690
(573) 751-4126 or (800) 726-7390

Montana

http://www.mt.gov/sao/polhldr.htm
126 North Sanders, Room 270
Helena, MT 59620
(406) 444-2040 or (800) 332-6148

Nebraska

http://www.nol.org/home/NDOI/
941 "O" Street, Suite 400
Lincoln, NE 68508-3690
(402) 471-2201 or (800) 833-0920

Nevada

http://www.state.nv.us/b&i/id/
1665 Hot Springs Road, Suite 152
Carson City, NV 89706-0646
(702) 687-4270 or (888) 872-3234

New Hampshire

http://www.state.nh.us/insurance/
169 Manchester St., Suite 1
Concord, NH 03301-5151
(603) 271-2261 or (800) 852-3416

New Jersey

http://www.naic.org/nj/div_ins.htm
20 West State Street
P.O. Box CN 329
Trenton, NJ 08625-0329
(609) 292-5316

New Mexico

PERA Building, 500 Old Santa Fe Trail
Santa Fe, NM 87501
(505) 827-4601 or (800) 947-4722

New York

http://www.ins.state.ny.us/nyins.htm
Empire State Plaza, Agency Building No. 1
Albany, NY 12257
(518) 474-6600 or (800) 342-3736

North Carolina

http://www.doi.state.nc.us/
P.O. Box 26387
Raleigh, NC 27611
(919) 733-7343

North Dakota

http://www.state.nd.us/ndins/
600 East Blvd., Dept. 401
Bismarck, ND 58505-0320
(701) 328-2440 or (800) 247-0560

Ohio

http://www.state.oh.us/ins/
2100 Stella Court
Columbus, OH 43215-1067
(614) 644-2658 or (800) 686-1526

Oklahoma

http://www.oid.state.ok.us/
3814 N. Santa Fe
P.O. Box 53408
Oklahoma City, OK 73118
(405) 521-2828 or (800) 522-0071

Oregon

http://www.cbs.state.or.us/external/ins/index.html
350 Winter St. NE, Room 200
Salem, OR 97310-0200
(503) 947-7980

Pennsylvania

http://www.state.pa.us/
1326 Strawberry Square
Harrisburg, PA 17120
(717) 787-2317 or (877) 881-6388

Rhode Island

233 Richmond St., Suite 233
Providence, RI 02903-4233
(401) 277-2223

South Carolina

http://www.state.sc.us/doi/
1612 Marion Street
P.O. Box 100105
Columbia, SC 29202-3105
(803) 737-6150 or (800) 768-3467

South Dakota

http://www.state.sd.us/state/executive/dcr/insurance/
118 W. Capitol
Pierre, SD 57501
(605) 773-3563

Tennessee

http://www.state.tn.us/commerce/insurdiv.html
Volunteer Plaza, 500 James Robertson Pkwy
Nashville, TN 37243-0565
(615) 741-2241 or (800) 342-4029

Texas

http://www.tdi.state.tx.us/
333 Guadalupe St.
Austin, TX 78701
(512) 463-6464 or (800) 252-3439

Utah

http://www.ins-dept.state.ut.us/
3110 State Office Building
Salt Lake City, UT 84114
(801) 538-3805 or (800) 439-3805

Vermont

http://www.state.vt.us/bis/
89 Main St., Drawer 20
Montpelier, VT 05620-3101
(802) 828-3301 or (800) 631-7788

Virginia

http://www.state.va.us/scc/division/boi/index.htm
P.O. Box 1157
Richmond, VA 23218
(804) 371-9741 or (800) 552-7945

Washington

http://www.wa.gov/ins/
14th Ave. & Water Street, Insurance Building
Olympia, WA 98504
(360) 753-7300 or (800) 562-6900

West Virginia

http://www.state.wv.us/insurance/
P.O. Box 50540
1124 Smith Street, Room 403
Charleston, WV 25305-0540
(304) 558-3386 or (800) 642-9004

Wisconsin

http://badger.state.wi.us/agencies/oci/oci_home.htm
121 East Wilson Street
Madison, WI 53702
(608) 266-3585 or (800) 236-8517

Wyoming

122 West 25th Street, 3rd Floor East
Cheyenne, WY 82002-0440
(307) 777-7401

For ERISA Plans

U.S. Department of Labor
Division of Technical Assistance and Inquiries
200 Constitution Ave., NW, Room N-5619
Washington, DC 20210
(202) 219-8776

Additional Resources

NCQA

National Committee for Quality Assurance
2000 L Street, NW, Suite 500
Washington, DC 20036
(202) 955-3500
www.ncqa.org

Consumer Advocacy & Resource Groups

Families USA
1334 G Street, NW
Washington, DC 20005
(202) 628-3030
www.familiesusa.org/managedcare/

National Coalition of Mental Health Professionals
and Consumers, Inc.
P.O. Box 438
Commack, NY 11725
(888) 729-6662 or (516) 424-5232
www.NoManagedCare.org/

HARP (Health Administration Responsibility
Project)
552 12th St.
Santa Monica, CA 90402-2908
www.harp.org/

Bazelon Center for Mental Health Law:
1101 15th Street, NW, Suite 1212
Washington, DC 20005-5002
(202) 467-5730
www.bazelon.org/

National Mental Health Association (NMHA)
1021 Prince Street
Alexandria, VA 22314-2971
(703) 684-7722
http://www.nmha.org

Statistical Analysis of Utilization Data

Milliman & Robertson
1301 Fifth Avenue, Suite 3800
Seattle, WA 98101

Practice Guidelines

Practice Guideline Coalition
www.unr.edu/psych/pgc/
National Guideline Clearinghouse www.guideline.gov
Medscape Psychiatry Practice Guidelines:
    http://psychiatry.medscape.com/Home/Topics
    /psychiatry/directories/dir-PSY
    .PracticeGuide.html

Publications

Psychotherapy Finances
13901 U.S. Highway 1, Suite 5
Juno Beach, FL 33408
(800) 869-8450
www.psyfin.com

Practice Strategies

American Association for Marriage & Family
Therapy
1133 15th St. NW
Suite 300
Washington, DC 20005-2710
(202)452-0109

Behavioral Healthcare Tomorrow
Manisses Communications Group, Inc.
P.O. Box 9758
Providence, RI 02940-9758

EAP Digest
Performance Resource Press, Inc.
1270 Rankin Drive
Suite F
Troy, MI 48083-2843

Managed Care Companies' Utilization Review Criteria

Magellan: www.magellanassist.com (Employer
    division; EAPs); www.magellanhealth.com
    (Health plans, HMOs, state Medicaid)
ValueOptions: www.valueoptions.com
United Behavioral Health: www.provweb.com

HMO/Insurance Enrollment Data

Interstudy Publications
P.O. Box 4366
St. Paul, MN 55104
(800) 844-3351
www.hmodata.com

Internet Billing, Claims and Fees Resources

HCFA = Health Care Financing Administration
    www.hcfa.gov.
ICD-9 & CPT codes = American Medical Association
    www.ama-assn.org/ or (800) 621-8335
Mental Health Practice Management Network
    www.casualforums.com/directory/mhpm/index.cgi
Therapist Insurer Profiling
    http://www.mentalhealth-madison.com
    /Documents/Rate_the_Insurer.htm

Bibliography

American Managed Behavioral Healthcare Association. (1997). *Any willing provider* [AMBHA position paper]. Washington, DC: Author.

American Psychiatric Association. (1994). *Diagnostic and statistical manual* (4th ed.). Washington, DC: Author.

Astrachan, B., Essock, S., Kahn, R., Masi, D., McLean, A., & Visotsky, H. (1995, July). The role of a payor advisory board in managed mental health care: The IBM approach. *Administration and Policy in Mental Health, 22*(6), 581.

Atkins, R. (1998, August). Stop managing care: Start managing financial risk. *Open Minds, 10*(4), 4.

Bengen-Seltzer, B. (1998, May). MCC is putting its money where its outcomes are. *Behavioral Health Outcomes, 3*(5), 1.

Bernstein, B.E., & Hartsell, T.L. (1998). *The portable lawyer for mental health professionals.* New York: Wiley.

Browning, C.H., & Browning, B.J. (1996). *How to partner with managed care.* New York: Wiley.

Dubin, W., & O'Brien, S. (1999, January). Quality management as a strategy for utilization management: Using statistical process control to manage the care of high risk patients. *Open Minds, 10*(9), 4.

Grace, M. (1999, April 14). State judge rejects claim against CHP. *Albany Times Union,* 13–73.

Grinfeld, M.J. (1999, March). Lawsuits break health plans grip: Are reforms imminent? *Psychiatric Times, 16*(3). http://www.mhsource.com/edu/psytimes/p990301a.html

Grinfeld, M.J. (1998, February). ERISA may shield HMO liability: Texas law under fire. *Psychiatric Times.* http://www.mhsource.com/edu/psytimes/p980252a.html

Hay Group. (1998). Health care plan design and cost trends—1988 through 1997. http://www.naphs.org/News/HayGroupReport.html

Hering, N. (1999, May). The erosion of confidentiality by managed care. *The Coalition Report.* (National Coalition of Mental Health Professionals & Consumers, Inc. newsletter.)

Hofer, T.P., Hayward, R.A., Greenfield, S., Wanger, E.H., Kaplan, S.H., & Manning, W.G. (1999, June 9). The unreliability of individual physician "report cards" for assessing the costs and quality of care of a chronic disease. *Journal of the American Medical Association, 281*(22), 2098–2105.

Holstein, et al. vs. Green Spring, et al. (1998). Civil Action No 98 CV 2453 (NP), in the United States District Court for the District of New Jersey. http://www.managedcaresurvival.com/ClassAction.html

Jane Doe vs. Community Health Plan-Kaiser Corporation & Christen Adey. (1999). In the Supreme Court of Albany County, NY, Decision and Order Index #7342-97, RJI No. 01-97-052157. Decision of Justice Joseph C. Teresi, March 1, 1999.

Kahn-Kothman, A.M. (1998, December). Your rights after termination without cause. *Physician's News Digest.* http://www.medscape.com/PNDI/PND/1998/12.98/1298kahn/1298kahn.html

Managed Behavioral Health News. (1998a, January 29). Minnesota Blues moves UM decision-making under network providers' control. *Managed Behavioral Health News, 4*(5), 1.

Managed Behavioral Health News. (1998b, September 17). State performance measurements plans push for services in new realms. *Managed Behavioral Health News, 4*(33), 1.

Managed Care Strategies. (1998a, May). HAI says the future is here with its "real time" outcomes analysis. *Managed Care Strategies, 6*(5), 5.

Managed Care Strategies. (1998b, June). Minnesota Health Plan Uses "Withholds" to Lower Costs and Spread Risk to Providers. *Managed Care Strategies, 6*(6), 4.

Managed Care Strategies. (1998c, December). Profits under capitated contracts are sliding for health care providers. *Managed Care Strategies, 6*(12), 1.

Managed Care Strategies. (1998d, February). What do employers want from behavioral health care? *Managed Care Strategies, 6*(2), 8.

Managed Care Strategies. (1999a, March). New licensing obstacles loom for small EAP operators. *Managed Care Strategies, 7*(3), 3.

Managed Care Strategies. (1999b, April). Taking the pulse of behavioral health care as the marketplace consolidates. *Managed Care Strategies, 7*(4), 7.

Mihalik, G. (1998, April–June). Accreditation in managed behavioral health care: An interview with Mary Cesare-Murphy and Claire Sharda. *Journal of Healthcare Finance, 54.*

Miller, I. (1996, Summer). Committee for quality assurance (NCQA): Who is the watchdog's master? *The Independent Practitioner, 16*(3), 133.

Miller, I. (1999). *Supplement to collusive behavior in the managed care industry.* Unpublished draft/update of 1997 letter to Department of Justice.

Miller, I. (1999). *Standards for constructing and criteria for evaluating mental health service guidelines.* Draft, May 14, 1999.

Mills, M. (1997, September). U.S. has 114 behavioral health professionals per 100,000 population. *Open Minds, 11*(9), 12.

Moran, M. (1998, June). Managing care with outcome data: New hopes, new responsibilities. *Behavioral Healthcare Tomorrow, 7*(3), 21.

National Committee for Quality Assurance. (1998). *Standards for accreditation of managed behavioral healthcare organizations.* Washington, DC: Author.

National Committee for Quality Assurance. (2000). *Standards and surveyor guidelines for the accreditation of MBHOs.* Washington, DC: Author.

Open Minds. (1998, December). Mergers and acquisitions continue to change the industry. *Open Minds, 10*(8), 4.

Open Minds Advisor. (1999, July). Humana, Oxford and United Healthcare cooperate on physician credentialing. *Open Minds Advisor, 1*(7), 8.

Oss, M., & Clary, J. (1997). Mergers and acquisitions continue to change the industry. *Open Minds, 11*(12), 4.

Oss, M., & Clary, J. (1998, January). EAP's are evolving to meet changing employer needs. *Open Minds, 12*(1), 4.

Perez, R.A. (1996). *ERISA litigation fundamentals.* Health Administration Responsibility Project (HARP). http://www.harp.org/perez.htm

Plocica vs. NYLCare of Texas, et al. (1998). Cause #141-175780-98, in the District Court of Tarrant County, TX, 141st Judicial District. http://www.ljx.com/LJXfiles/hmo/plocica_cpt.html

Pomerantz, J.M. (1999a). Behavioral health matters: Clinical practice guidelines. *Drug Benefit Trends, 11*(4), 2.

Pomerantz, J.M. (1999b). Behavioral health matters: Is confidentiality still protected under managed behavioral health care? *Drug Benefit Trends, 11*(2), 2.

Pomerantz, J.M. (1999c). Behavioral health matters—The behavioral health war zone. *Drug Benefit Trends, 11*(1), 2.

Practice Strategies. (1998, August). Industry trends: Magellan focus is on systems, provider network. *Practice Strategies, 4*(8), 1.

Practice Strategies. (1999, March). More therapists offer EMDR, but will MCO's pay? *Practice Strategies, 5*(3), 1.

Practice Strategies. (1999, January). Stranded online. *Practice Strategies, 5*(1), 1.

Practice Strategies. (1999, September). Short on referrals? *Practice Strategies, 5*(9), 10.

Psychotherapy Finances. (1998, October). Managed care notes: Resist the impulse to claim expertise in too many specialty areas. *Psychotherapy Finances, 24*(10), 8.

Rabasca, L. (1998, November). APA pursues "test cases" to set legal precedents. *APA Monitor, 29*(11). http://www.apa.org/monitor/nov98/mc.html

Shore, K. (1997). *Don't let them take your mind and spirit: On being called a "provider."* National Coalition of Mental Health Professionals and Consumers. Commack, NY: Author. http://www.NoManagedCare.org/provider.html

ValueOptions. (1999). *Provider handbook: Clinical criteria.* Falls Church, VA: Author. http://www.valueoptions.com/providertoc.htm

Wrich, J.T. (1998). *Brief summary of audit findings of managed behavioral health care services.* Submitted to the Congressional Budget Office, revised March 1998.

Zieman, G. (1998). *The handbook of managed behavioral healthcare.* Tiburon, CA: Jossey-Bass.

Index